Succeeding in Your GPST Stage 2 Situational Judgement (SJT) / Professional Dilemmas Practice Questions for GPST / GPVTS Stage 2 Selection

Matt Green and Nicole Corriette

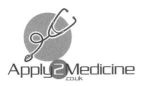

Published by Apply2 Ltd
Chelsea House
Chelsea Street
New Basford,
Nottingham, NG7 7HN
0800 6121135
www.Apply2Medicine.co.uk

A catalogue record for this title is available from the British Library

ISBN: 978–0–9556746–9–3

Typeset by RefineCatch Limited, Bungay
Printed by Bell and Bain, Glasgow

Contents

About the Authors

Dr Nicole Corriette MRCGP (Distinction) MBBS (Hons) BSc (Hons) DFSRH DRCOG DCH

Dr Nicole Corriette is originally from London and trained at University College London Medical School. She was awarded the University College and Middlesex Hospital Club Award for her achievements in pre-clinical medicine and also won the Smith-Kline and Beecham Prize Award for her achievements in her intercalated BSc. She graduated in 2003 with a Distinction in her MBBS and a First Class Intercalated BSc in Physiology. Following her love for general practice she joined a Pan-London VTS scheme in 2005 and completed her registrar year on the Barnet VTS. In 2007 she completed her MRCGP with a distinction overall, and was one of only 20 candidates that year to achieve a merit in all four components. Subsequently she was nominated for the Fraser Rose medal by the RCGP. She is currently a partner in a large practice in Dunstable and also helps deliver GPST courses for Apply2Medicine.

Matt Green BSc (Hons) MPhil

After completing his BSc in Biochemistry Matt went on to complete an MPhil at the Royal Marsden Hospital in London. This involved working closely with medical professionals on a number of projects developing novel drugs for the treatment of ovarian cancer. Since establishing Apply2Medicine in 2005 Matt has been supporting doctors to progress their career through providing application and interview advice together with helping doctors to develop their non-clinical skills including leadership, management, teaching and communication.

Acknowledgements

I would like to thank Dr Nigel Giam for showing me that with the correct teaching and training anything is possible. I would also like to thank my previous VTS course organiser Dr Sanjiv Ahluwalia for supporting me during my registrar year and reminding me that in the end being a GP is truly worth all the hard work.

I would like to say thank you to everyone who made this publication possible including the whole team at Apply2Medicine. Special thanks must go to Sarah Bell for all her hard efforts and sharing my vision of supporting doctors at every step of their career to become a reality.

Preface

Situational Judgement Tests (SJTs) or Professional Dilemmas form a significant part of the GPST recruitment process and yet many doctors will not have experienced questions of this type under formal examination conditions. It is therefore essential that candidates sitting the GPST Stage 2 exam have a clear understanding on how to approach questions of this type as poor performance in this section will almost certainly result in not progressing to the Stage 3 selection day.

This interactive book, which contains extensive guidance on how to approach the various types of scenarios you will face together with 70 practice questions (including detailed explanations of all the answers), is designed to help doctors prepare for and successfully complete their GPST Stage 2 exam.

On behalf of Nicole, Matt and Apply2Medicine we would like to take this opportunity to wish you the best of luck with your application to the GPST programme.

Chapter 1 Introduction to Situational Judgement Tests

Situational Judgement Tests (SJTs), which are sometimes referred to as Professional Dilemmas, are psychological tests that essentially present the candidate with a work-based situation and asks what he/she would do in that particular scenario. They are designed particularly to test your professional competencies and assess how you would act in hypothetical and challenging situations that you might encounter in the workplace. They are not a test of clinical knowledge, although some basic ethical principles are needed in order to answer some of the trickier questions! The answers should however, draw on the general knowledge and life experience you have acquired through medical school and as a life as a doctor.

Why use Situational Judgement Tests?
The first SJT was used in 1926 before being used extensively by psychologists in the US military during World War II. SJTs are now used by many organisations to identify suitable candidates for particular jobs, assessing whether their responses suit the particular role they are applying for. Thus the SJTs used in the GPST selection process are particularly designed to identify individuals who are suitable for a career in general practice. The SJTs you will be faced with are designed and written by general practitioners, and aim to identify the candidates who are likely to be more successful at the more intensive Stage 3 assessments. The questions are carefully designed and have been reviewed and statistically validated to ensure they test the required competencies.

Person Specification
The SJTs assess a variety of themes – from problem solving and decision making to interpersonal skills. To put it simply, the SJTs you will be sitting are designed to establish whether you have the qualities of a good GP. The questions are based on scenarios that you may encounter as a second year foundation doctor, and you need to answer them from that perspective. As the clinical knowledge component is tested in the MCQs/EMQS, they are fundamentally assessing whether you have the required personal skills that appear in the National Person Specification for the GP selection process (**http://www.gprecruitment.org.uk**) as well as fulfilling the duties of a doctor

as set out by the GMC. The personal skills they are looking for are as follows:

- **Empathy and Sensitivity:** Your competency and enthusiasm to take in the perspectives of others and whether you treat others with understanding. This involves handling situations sensitively and treating others as individuals as well as respecting patient's rights to confidentiality.
- **Communication Skills:** The capacity to adjust your behaviour and language to the needs of differing situations. Your ability to deal with individuals of all levels.
- **Conceptual Thinking and Problem Solving:** Your capability to think beyond the obvious, to analyse particular situations and to be flexible in forming an appropriate plan of action.
- **Coping with Pressure:** Your ability to recognise your own limitations and develop appropriate coping mechanisms for stressful and pressured situations.
- **Organisation and Planning:** Your capability to organise all resources (e.g. time/information/people) effectively in a planned manner. The ability to delegate effectively where appropriate.
- **Managing Others and Team Involvement:** Your capacity to work effectively in partnership with others.
- **Professional Integrity:** Your ability to be accountable for your own decisions and to act without delay if you have good reason to believe that you or a colleague may be putting patients at risk.
- **Learning and Personal Development:** Your eagerness to keep your knowledge and skills up to date and to learn from experience.

Visit **http://www.gprecruitment.org.uk** for more information on the above.

Situational Judgement Test Format

The SJT component for 2009 comprises of 50 questions which you need to complete in 115 minutes. The time available has been increased over previous years (last year in 2008 candidates only had 105 minutes). This gives you just over two minutes per question, (two minutes and 18 seconds to be precise), which in all honesty is not a lot of time. There are two different types of SJT question you may be asked and both formats are used in the actual exam. These are:

- Ranking questions
- Multiple action questions

In both questions they are looking for the most appropriate answers. However in the ranking questions you need to rank your answers from most appropriate to the least appropriate. On the other hand, in the multiple action questions you need to choose the two or three most appropriate actions from a list of five or seven options respectively. You do not need to justify your answers in either of the types of question.

Ranking Questions

In these questions you are given a particular scenario with approximately four or five possible actions which you need to rank from the most appropriate action to the least appropriate action. There are no tied rankings in these questions.

An example of such a question may be:

> *Upon joining a MDT team as an ST1 doctor you suspect that a senior nurse within the team is stealing prescription drugs and possibly self medicating. On closer observation you actually see the nurse steal the drugs from the cabinet at the beginning the shift prior to her conducting a ward round.*

Rank in order from 1 to 5 the following actions in response to this situation, where 1 is the most appropriate action and 5 is the least appropriate action.

   A. You ignore what you have just seen. You have only been a member of the team for a matter of weeks and do not want to interfere.
   B. You ask to discuss with the nurse immediately your concerns away from the ward, ensure that they do not have any further contact with patients and encourage them to go home.
   C. Attempt to seek the opinion of your Registrar but find that he is unavailable for the next hour.
   D. You decide to raise the issue at your next appraisal to ensure that the nurse receives help.
   E. You report the matter as a critical incident as per your Trust's protocol.

The answer to this question will be discussed later in Chapter 3 where we will go through some worked examples.

Multiple Action Questions

In this format you will be faced with a particular scenario that usually poses some sort of problem or dilemma. You are then presented with between five to seven possible actions and need to select either two or the three of most suitable options. You do not need to rank the options chosen or place them in any particular order.

An example of a question in this format would be:

> *You are nearing the end of a busy shift when one of your patient's family members confronts you in the middle of the ward in a very aggressive manner regarding the standard of care their relative is receiving. You are not familiar with the patient's progress and need to leave promptly as you have an outside engagement.*

Choose the 3 most appropriate actions to take out of the 7 actions below (no need to order).

A.   See if one of your colleagues who has just started their shift and has been directly involved in the treatment of the patient is available to update the relative.

B.   Request that one of the nurses addresses the situation on your behalf.

C.   Calm the relative down and assure them that you are going to personally look into their concerns.

D.   Request one of your nurse colleagues to escort the relative to a consultation room to await a member of staff who can discuss their concerns.

E.   Address the situation there and then and advise the relative that they have nothing to worry about.

F.   Tell the relative that you have not been involved in the care of the patient and that they should ring the ward tomorrow morning to raise their concerns.

G.   Tell the relative that you are not on the ward and that they should raise their concerns with someone else.

Again the answer to this question will be discussed later in Chapter 3.

Suggested Approach to answering the questions

As stated previously you will have just over two minutes to answer each question and effective time management is therefore crucial. The ranking questions typically take slightly more thought and thus you may need to spend slightly longer thinking about these than the multiple action questions. As a rule do not spend too long reading through the question and possible actions, as you will need to analyse the situation and think hard about the options before answering.

Therefore, if possible, do not read the question and answer stems more than twice. However, it is useful when reading the question to get a feel for a summary of what the dilemma is e.g. Is it a patient safety issue? Is it confidentiality issue? This is, as you will discover in the later chapters, because many of the popular topics asked follow a set structure in how to answer the questions. Simply put, the scenarios may change but the way you deal with the underlying issue is repetitive for a lot of the questions, and thus it is possible to structure your approach.

For most of the questions there will be an action or actions that are obviously the most appropriate or least appropriate. It is useful to eliminate these first and then use your analytical thinking to rank the remaining options. The important thing is to use your instinct initially and eliminate the most or least obvious options. SJTs are designed to test your natural instincts so try not to over analyse the question. The first impression is usually the correct one. There are a few options that appear difficult, but with practise you will learn how to spot these options and deal with them correctly. In general, the multiple action questions are a lot more straightforward as the most appropriate actions are usually quite obvious. However, you may get a multiple action question where all the answers are appropriate or inappropriate. Here you will need to look at all the actions and choose the best two or three actions, which may mean picking the best of a bad bunch. Thus you need to read all the options you are provided with before deciding which ones are the most appropriate actions to take. It is also important to confirm that collectively your answers do not contradict each other.

Finally, remember that these situations are designed to simulate real life situations that you may be in. Thus you need to answer them from the perspective of a second year foundation doctor. One of the most important points about being a junior doctor is trying to achieve a balance between recognising when you are out of your depth, but at the same time not shirking responsibility when it is a situation you should be trained to deal with.

Therefore, when answering the questions, don't be afraid to ask for help from senior colleagues if you are uncomfortable with the situation. However, when dealing with a common scenario in a foundation doctor's day, show the examiner that you are willing to accept responsibility and do not immediately pass the responsibility to others. Again this will become clearer as you go through the practice questions.

Scoring of Situational Judgement Tests

There are different numbers of marks available depending on the types of questions asked. Some questions only require you to choose two options and other harder questions require the ranking of five options which means the maximum number of marks per question varies. In the 2008 exam there were between 10 and 20 points available for a question, and the maximum number of marks you could score for the whole paper was 782, which illustrates that answers for each of the 50 questions are awarded different marks. To score the maximum number of marks available for a question you need to answer the question in exactly the same way as a 'model answer', i.e. the answer that the examiners feel is the most appropriate and that fits closest with the desired qualities they are testing.

However, as the SJTs are testing personal skills and attributes it would be difficult to only mark them based on one single correct answer. We are all individuals and may have appropriate responses to a situation which may differ from those of others. Thus the questions are not just simply marking you on whether you are right or wrong. They are looking at how your answer compares to the model answer. The closest your answer is to the model answer the more marks you will score. If your answer is similar to the model answer, but perhaps you have ranked two items slightly differently, you will still receive a high number of marks as long as your answer as a whole is appropriate. Indeed, for some questions there are different responses which are very similar but both ways could be deemed appropriate at the same ranking. If your answer has little or nothing in common with the model answer you will score little or even zero marks. If you rank something completely inappropriate as the most appropriate answer, or vice versa, you are also likely to score very little marks. For example, if you prioritise answering a phone call over a collapsed patient on the ward, you are likely to score less, regardless of your other rankings! Thankfully, the most obvious or least obvious answers are usually, but not always, the easiest to rank.

It should be mentioned however, that when answering the multiple action questions, you have less room to differ from the model answer if you want to score full marks. This is because you are asked to only select two or three most appropriate options. In most questions of this type, the two or three correct options are really the only appropriate actions to take. Thus if you choose two or three completely different options to the model answer, they are unlikely to be suitable. Obviously, if only one of your answers is different to the model answer, you will get marks for getting the other options correct. Again you will understand this more as you work through the practice questions in this book.

It should be noted, however, that for the purpose of this book it would not be practical to give you every possible partial mark answer when going through the practice questions. We will however give you a partial mark variant that is the closest to the model answer and that would give you the highest number of marks. Obviously the further your answer is from the model answer or the alternative partial mark answer the less marks you are likely to score.

Scores required for short-listing

The scores required for short-listing will vary from year to year and will depend on the number and the quality of the candidates completing the exam. Typically they divide the total scores into four bands, with Band 4 comprising the candidates with the highest marks and Band 1 being the lowest. Last year, a score in Band 2 or above was required to be short-listed. However, some deaneries may be highly competitive and you may need a higher score to proceed to Stage 3.

As previously stated, in 2008 the maximum marks you could score in the SJT component was 782. The highest score actually achieved by a candidate last year was 714 and the minimum score was 256. The mean score, you will be pleased to hear, was 645. Last year, this score would have been a Band 3, and as most of the candidates fell into this band, most of the candidates would have been short-listed (see table). This again re-iterates that you do not need to answer every single question precisely as determined by the model answer to be short-listed.

The table below gives you some idea of the marks scored and the percentage of people who fell into each band in the 2008 SJT component. This can also be found on the GP Recruitment website (**http://www.gprecruitment.org.uk**).

Band	Approximate Percentage in Band	Score Range Professional Dilemmas
Band 1	8%	256–597
Band 2	19%	598–629
Band 3	58%	630–682
Band 4	13%	683–714

As you can see, in 2008 only 8 per cent of candidates fell below Band 2 and were unsuccessful as these candidates were unlikely to be suited for a career in general practice. However, although the test is designed specifically to sieve out those of you who naturally fit the person specifications required for general practice, with preparation one can learn how to train yourself to think like the examiners and come up with the model answer or something close!

You will have the chance to practise some worked examples first to familiarise yourself with the types of questions you will face before you tackle the practice questions later in this book! You will also find detailed explanations of what the model answers are together with what deviations in the answers would be acceptable to score partial marks.

However, before we even get to that stage, let's go on to discuss some of the common questions you may be asked in the exam and provide you with background information on various areas that will aid you in your preparations.

Chapter 2 Common Questions in the SJTs

Although SJTs are designed to assess a candidate's personal skills and not academic knowledge they do however assess your work-based knowledge. This work-based knowledge involves being aware of certain rules and regulations that we practise on a daily basis, most of the time without even realising. For example, it may be common sense to deal with an upset patient before checking your emails, but perhaps that is because we are taught that we must always make the care of the patient our top priority. Our code of practice is largely set out by guidance from the GMC, and as stated before, in order to meet the requirements for general practice you need to fulfil the GMC criteria of a 'good doctor'. Thus it is useful to know some of the common topics that come up in the exam and the specific GMC guidance relating to it.

In addition, you will find that for each section of the person specification you are assessed on there are recurring themes in the sort of scenarios you will be asked asked. For example, there may be a variety of different scenarios which each assess how you would deal with confidentiality issues. In general, although the scenarios are different there is a correct way to answer these questions, which is much easier if you actually know the basic ethical principles surrounding the dilemma. This will become clearer as you go through the practice questions but it is useful to have an clear understanding of some of the key ethical dilemmas you may come across and the correct approach to dealing with them.

In this chapter we will discuss some of the common topics that are asked in the exam and then go on to provide you with detailed guidance on some of the ethical principles behind the questions where appropriate.

Common Questions in the SJTs

Patient safety issues

This is a very common theme present in many of the questions. Examples of such questions include an underperforming colleague or situations involving near misses or critical events. Patient safety must always come first and you must always assess whether there is an immediate or potential patient safety issue in the question asked. In such questions, any patient safety issues must always be your first priority. Any near misses or critical events must never be ignored and must always be reported.

In general, if you are faced with a question where a patient's safety has been compromised you must always take steps to immediately safeguard the patient and prevent any further safety breaches. Thus any options which involve immediately dealing with the situation must be ranked first. You also have a duty to try and investigate why the event occurred and take steps to prevent it from happening, but this can be done after the risk to the patient has been removed or diminished, and these options should be prioritised as less urgent. For example if you were provided with a scenario where a patient was given too much morphine, your immediate priority would be to stabilise the patient before filling in an incident form.

Ethical Guidance on Patient Safety

The ethical guidance behind patient safety is taken from the GMC guidance in 'Good Medical Practice' (paragraph 6) which states:

> 'If you have good reason to think that patient safety is or may be seriously compromised by inadequate premises, equipment, or other resources, policies or systems, you should put the matter right if that is possible. In all other cases you should draw the matter to the attention of your employing or contracting body. If they do not take adequate action, you should take independent advice on how to take the matter further. You must record your concerns and the steps you have taken to try to and resolve them'

Thus if you have any concerns at all about the safety of your patient you have a duty to deal with the issue at hand yourself or if not possible involve someone else who is capable of doing so. This guidance is tied in very closely with the guidance on dealing with underperforming colleagues which is also a very common theme. Here you may also need to involve someone more senior if you feel patient safety is compromised and you feel ill equipped to deal with the matter yourself. We will now go on to discuss that issue.

Issues with the work ethics of colleagues

These situations may vary from a colleague attending work late to one where you may need to inform others about an underperforming colleague (whistle blowing). In these situations, you need to determine if there is indeed an issue at hand that needs to be addressed. This may not be clear cut and when deciding this you must consider whether there is or potentially could be a patient safety issue, as this can never be ignored. For example, if a colleague is five minutes late for their shift it may not warrant serious action or any action at all, compared to a colleague that is consistently two hours late as this may put patients at risk through lack of cover.

However, if you decide there is indeed an issue, you then need to decide whether the situation needs to be dealt with immediately or if it can be postponed to a later time, which may be more appropriate depending on the circumstance. However, any issues where patients may be at risk must always be dealt with immediately. Thus although it may be appropriate to speak to a colleague privately after work about a personal issue it would not be appropriate to delay dealing with the matter if he had turned up to work drunk. You will also need to decide whether you feel comfortable in handling the situation yourself or whether you need to seek advice from a senior colleague.

You should also try to avoid prioritising any actions that involve directly criticising or confronting colleagues or actions where you make accusations with little evidence. However, if it is appropriate to speak to your colleague sensitively about a given matter because it is not a serious offence, you should try to do this before involving other colleagues such as your Registrar or Consultant. This may be the case when a colleague is consistently late (but only by five minutes) for their shift for example. In this situation you may be able to just have a quiet word with them about the situation. This would be more suitable than going to your Consultant immediately or chastising them regarding their lateness when you have no idea about the reasons behind it.

Therefore for these types of questions you need to decide how severe the issue at hand is and whether you need to involve anyone else or whether a simple word to the person in question will suffice. Although you do have a duty to protect your patients, you must always remember to be sensitive in your approach when dealing with your work colleagues and try to minimise any adverse outcomes from the situation if possible.

Ethical guidance on conduct and performance issues of colleagues

The definition of a 'whistle blower' is a person within an organisation who exposes misconduct or malpractice to a person capable of taking corrective action. It is your professional duty as a doctor to recognise if there is a problem which compromises patient safety and never ignore it. However, it is not always your responsibility to deal entirely with the matter by yourself. Thus you may need to inform a more senior colleague of the problem if you feel it is out of your depth to deal with it alone.

The GMC provides specific guidance within the Good Medical Practice guide which addresses the issues of conduct and performance issues in colleagues in paragraphs 43 to 45. In general, you need to be able to recognise the problem and be able to assess whether you will tackle the problem by yourself or involve others. This can be quite awkward and you need to recognise your own limitations and whether it is a situation you can comfortably deal with. It is professional courtesy in most cases to be sympathetic and try to deal with the matter locally (e.g. discuss with your Registrar/Consultant) before involving larger agencies such as the GMC, which should be the last resort. In making your decisions you must make appropriate conclusions on whom to involve e.g. informing relevant people including your Consultant as opposed to gossiping with the nursing staff. You should also start lower down the hierarchy when discussing other colleagues locally within the hospital through discussing the matter with your Registrar or Consultant before approaching the Clinical Director of the hospital.

However, there may be cases which are not resolved by, for example your Consultant ignoring the problem. In this case you may need to contact someone more senior such as the Clinical Director, or go to an outside authority, for example the PCT or GMC. You must never ignore the problem if patient safety is compromised as stated by the GMC in paragraph 6 of 'Good Medical Practice'.

Criminal Issues

Examples of such questions may include a situation where a colleague is viewing child pornography or there is a theft from the ward. As a rule, when answering any of these questions you must always have your facts completely straight before addressing the situation, especially if it may involve incriminating another colleague or patient. Thus it is sensible to prioritise answers that involve establishing the facts about what has happened first before confronting anyone or involving anyone else.

You should also prioritise any actions that involve immediately dealing with the situation, and leave actions such as incident forms and preventative measures until later. You must also be able to use your common sense to assess the severity of the crime and use your judgement in when to involve more senior authorities. For example, although all theft is illegal it may not be necessary to involve the police for a minor theft, and thus you must show that you are able to apply common sense to individual situations.

However, if the criminal issue compromises patient safety or if it involves the work ethic of a colleague, it may become necessary to involve someone more senior and escalate the matter to a higher level. This may be the case in a scenario where a colleague is stealing prescription drugs or viewing child pornography, as obviously patients may be at risk in these cases. Here you may need to involve your Consultant or even the Clinical Director or GMC if the matter is not dealt with. The ethical principles behind this approach involve the same ethics previously discussed with regards to patient safety and poorly performing colleagues i.e. you must always safeguard your patients.

Finally you must also use your common sense in deciphering which senior authority to inform first. Although there may be a criminal issue at hand and the police may need to be involved at some point, you are only a foundation doctor, and thus it may be sensible to go to your Registrar or Consultant first before contacting the police yourself. As previously stated, it is common courtesy when dealing with conduct issues in colleagues to deal with the matter locally first. Thus it is perfectly acceptable to discuss the matter with your Registrar or Consultant who can then call the police if necessary. In general, when answering these types of questions, contacting the police should be prioritised after involving someone senior within the hospital to deal with the matter.

Confidentiality Issues

This is a common theme and questions may involve anything from dealing with a family member translating for a patient, to situations where you are asked to keep information out of a patient's notes. Questions surrounding having to inform the DVLA about a patient driving against medical advice are also common. You must be well aware of the situations where you are allowed to break confidentiality, but must always attempt to maintain patient confidentiality where possible. As a rule if you do need to break confidentiality, it should always be the last resort when other measures have failed. Also, you must always inform the patient that you are breaking their confidentiality and for what reasons prior to actually doing so.

Ethical Guidance on Confidentiality

You must respect patient's rights to confidentiality. The GMC states that patients have a right to expect that information about them will be held in confidence by their doctors. There may be a few difficult scenarios in the exam where you are asked if it is acceptable to breach confidentiality or where you are dealing with confidentiality of a minor. The GMC sets out clear guidance about when confidentiality can be breached. There are six main areas where confidentiality can be breached, however, the four most common areas you may come across are:

- If the patient consents to the disclosure of the information.
- If the disclosure is required by law e.g. notification of a suspected communicable disease.
- If you are ordered to disclose information by a judge or presiding officer of a court.
- Where the benefits to an individual or to society of the disclosure outweigh the public and the patient's interest in keeping the information confidential. This may be justified if it is in the public's or patient's interest and failure to do so may expose the patient or others to risk of death or serious harm.

In all cases where you consider disclosing information without consent from the patient, you must weigh the possible harm (both to the patient, and the overall trust between doctors and patients) against the benefits which are likely to arise from the release of information. This may include informing the DVLA about a person who is driving against medical advice (see later) or an HIV-positive person who knowingly has unprotected sex with his partner who is unaware of their HIV status. It may also include child protection or elderly protection issues.

Confidentiality and Children

You have the same duty of confidentiality to children and young people as you have to adults. This means that you should have the child's consent to share any necessary information with others, as you would do for an adult. However, prior to this you need to assess whether the child has the capacity to consent. The GMC states that this is essentially the same as assessing capacity in adults and you need to assess that they are able to:

> 'Understand the nature, risk and benefits of any investigations or treatments you propose, as well as the consequences of not having treatment'.

This is often also known as 'Gillick Competence'. If the child is competent then the grounds for breaking confidentiality are the same as that in adults.

If the child is not competent or lacks capacity to consent, and declines for you to share the information, then the following rules from the GMC apply.

'Occasionally, children who lack the capacity to consent will share information with you on the understanding that their parents are not informed. You should usually try to persuade the child to involve a parent in such circumstances. If they refuse and you consider it is necessary and in the child's best interests for the information to be shared (for example, to enable a parent to make an important decision, or to provide proper care for the child), you can disclose information to parents or appropriate authorities. You should record your discussions and reasons for sharing the information'.

Thus in general, do not forget that minors have the same rights to confidentiality as adults. However, be aware that you may need to break their confidentiality in exceptional circumstances, and this may include informing their parents.

Confidentiality and the DVLA

As previously stated questions involving breaking confidentiality to the DVLA are very common and thus it is useful to know the rules that the DVLA and GMC have set out involving breaching confidentiality in this area. The guidance issued by the GMC is as below:

'It is the duty of the licence holder or licence applicant to notify DVLA of any medical condition, which may affect safe driving. On occasions however, there are circumstances in which the licence holder cannot, or will not do so.'

The GMC has issued clear guidelines applicable to such circumstances, which state:

- The DVLA is legally responsible for deciding if a person is medically unfit to drive. They need to know when driving licence holders have a condition, which may, now or in the future, affect their safety as a driver.
- Therefore, where patients have such conditions, you should:
  - Make sure that the patients understand that the condition may impair their ability to drive. If a patient is incapable of understanding this advice, for example because of dementia, you should inform the DVLA immediately.
  - Explain to patients that they have a legal duty to inform the DVLA about the condition.
- If the patients refuse to accept the diagnosis or the effect of the condition on their ability to drive, you can suggest that the patients seek a second medical opinion, and make appropriate arrangements for the patients to do so. You should advise patients not to drive until the second opinion has been obtained.

- If patients continue to drive when they are not fit to do so, you should make every reasonable effort to persuade them to stop. This may include telling their next of kin, if they agree you may do so.
- If you do not manage to persuade patients to stop driving, or you are given or find evidence that a patient is continuing to drive contrary to advice, you should disclose relevant medical information immediately, in confidence, to the medical adviser at the DVLA.
- Before giving information to the DVLA you should inform the patient of your decision to do so. Once the DVLA has been informed, you should also write to the patient, to confirm that a disclosure has been made.

Thus to summarise, although it is the patient's duty to inform the DVLA if they are unfit to drive, there may be situations where they refuse to follow your advice. By continuing to drive they may be putting the public at risk and therefore you may need to break confidentiality and would be allowed to do so. However, as stated before this should be the last resort and you should make every attempt to stop the patient from driving before doing so. This may include offering them a second opinion or discussing it with their next of kin if they consent for you to do so.

Child protection issues

Examples of such questions could include situations where minors are having under age sex or incidences of domestic violence involving children. As a rule the needs of the child are paramount and you must be prepared to break confidentiality if you feel a child's welfare is in danger. You must never ignore a child protection issue and must always put the needs of the child first, even before the needs of the parent.

Ethical Guidance on Child Protection

Child protection is a key topic and you must be aware of the basic rules relating to it. If there are any child protection issues in a SJT you must deal with them promptly and correctly. The needs of the child are always paramount and you are allowed to break confidentiality if you feel a child is in danger, for example by informing social services about domestic violence occurring in a household if you are concerned a child is at risk. Again it is advised that you inform the parent of the need to break confidentiality.

However, there may be more difficult cases where you need to break confidentiality against the wishes of the child. Although, anyone over the age of

16 is automatically assumed to be able to give consent and has the same confidentiality rights as an adult, anyone under the age of 18 is still a minor and any harm done to that person is still considered child protection. Thus you may need to break confidentiality in circumstances of this nature. For example when a 16 year old girl is being assaulted by her partner, even if she asks you not to do so. This is distinctly different to an over 18 year old being domestically abused where you would need to have good grounds, e.g. concerns over the welfare of any children or immediate concerns for her safety, to go and break her confidentiality and inform others against her wishes.

Under age sex is also common and when dealing with this situation you need to assess whether any under 16 year old is 'Gillick Competent' and able to understand the implications of sexual intercourse to be able to give their consent. Thus although it is technically illegal to have sex under the age of 16 it may not always be necessary to break confidentiality and inform anyone else if you have no concerns of any coercion. Thus if you have a mature 15 year old who is having consensual sex with her 17 year old boyfriend, you do not need to necessarily involve her parents, police or social services. Thus you need to apply common sense and judgement to the situation.

However, it is important to remember that anyone under the age of 13 is not considered mature enough to give their consent for a sexual relationship. Therefore it is considered rape if anyone under 13 years of age is involved in any sexual activity. Thus you must inform social services if anyone aged under thirteen is having sex regardless of the age of their partner, and regardless of whether they consent for you to do so.

Probity

Questions on probity are designed to assess your personal and professional integrity and can range from questions about accepting gifts from patients to situations where you are asked to lie or withhold the truth e.g. you are asked to lie on an insurance form or withhold some necessary legal information. Accepting gifts from patients is discussed in more detail shortly, but you must always act with honesty and integrity in all situations. You must not lie to your patients nor lie on any legal documents including insurance forms as you will be in breach of this guidance and indeed the law with the latter.

It is also not best practice to lie to your colleagues even if you feel you have a good reason. You may encounter questions where you are asked to make up an excuse to a patient or a colleague and these particular actions in general should be prioritised as being inappropriate. They may not however always be the most inappropriate action. For example, if you are asked to deal with a clinical situation you are not comfortable in dealing with, it may be more appropriate to make up an excuse to get out of it rather than dealing with it incorrectly and putting a patient at risk. However, you should not prioritise lying over telling your colleague the truth, which in this situation may mean admitting your lack of experience.

You must also never abuse the doctor-patient relationship and use it to your advantage. For example, using your position as a professional and encouraging patients to give you money or gifts, or forming sexual relationships with your patients when they are in a vulnerable position, is wrong and would be abusing your position as a doctor.

Ethical Guidance on Accepting Gifts from Patients

This is a common ethical dilemma that arises in SJTs and may pose itself as a question where a patient may present you with a gift for example money or a bottle of alcohol. The GMC guidance contained within 'Good Medical Practice' is that 'You must not encourage patients to give, lend or bequeath money or gifts that will directly or indirectly benefit you'. However, the confusing issue is that this does not necessarily mean you cannot accept gifts. There is no generic answer to a question surrounding gifts but you can apply some general rules. Firstly, you must try and assess whether the gift is appropriate for the service you have offered e.g. a box of chocolates for providing palliative care to a relative may raise less suspicion than being given £100 for taking blood from a patient. You must also make sure that the patient is aware that there is no need to give you a gift to receive good medical care. However, you must also try not to offend the patient by declining a simple appropriate gift, as this may affect the doctor-patient relationship. When declining a gift that you feel inappropriate, you must give a reasonable and sensitive explanation to the patient. You may also accept the gift if appropriate, but you must try to ensure that the patient understands that they are under no obligation to keep giving you gifts. This will become clearer as you begin to complete the practice questions later in this book.

Arranging cover issues

Examples of these questions involve issues where you are about to go off duty and there is no one to cover or issues surrounding hand over e.g. can you hand over to your Consultant if there is no one else available or should you stay till cover arrives? In general you must always ensure before going off duty that there is no risk to your patients' safety. If there is no cover available the patients will obviously be at risk, and you must not simply leave at the end of your shift or leave without handing over. However, on the other hand if you were to then go on to cover a shift when you have been working all day and are exhausted you may also be putting a patient's safety at risk by doing so. Thus these questions may be quite difficult and confusing. The key to answering these questions is to ensure that the patient's safety is not compromised at all even if that means handing over to someone like your Consultant if you are unsafe to continue your shift!

Ethical Guidance on Cover

Again there is specific GMC guidance contained within 'Good Medical Practice' (paragraph 48) which states:

> *'You must be satisfied that, when you are off duty, suitable arrangements have been made for your patients' medical care. These arrangements should include effective handover procedures, involving clear communication with healthcare colleagues. If you are concerned that the arrangements are not suitable, you should take steps to safeguard patient care and you must follow the guidance in paragraph 6 (patient safety paragraph – see before)'*

Thus you cannot simply leave your shift without ensuring that there are adequate measures and resources to ensure the safety of your patients. You must also never leave your shift without handing over correctly, and to the appropriate person e.g. a fellow doctor as opposed to a nurse. If you are concerned about the arrangements for cover, e.g. if you are asked to cover a night shift when you have just done the day shift, you must raise this issue with the correct person and not ignore the matter. Again this will become more apparent as you complete the practice questions.

Work/life balance questions

This sort of question usually takes place in the form that you are asked to stay late on your shift when you have made other plans or something to that effect. The key to answering these questions is to think about patient safety. You must deal with any life threatening patient issues before leaving your shift but at the same time you are entitled to have a personal life and outside commitments. Obviously, it is not suitable to just forget about your duty of care to your patients and compromise their safety by attending to your other commitments. However in most cases there will be some sort of compromise where you will be able to delegate tasks in order to achieve a work/life balance. As the examiners are looking for candidates that can demonstrate that they can achieve this balance, you must aim to show this in your answer to these types of questions.

Therefore if you are given a scenario where you are asked to cover a shift on your day off when you have plans for example, do not immediately volunteer if there are other actions that would ensure patient safety together with you being able to have your day off. You will not score points for being so devoted to work that you cannot demonstrate the ability to balance both your work and personal life. This will lead to burnout and is not a healthy trait!

Therefore the key to answering these questions is to know which tasks can be delegated/postponed and which ones needs to be dealt with immediately. Obviously, any patient safety issues need to be addressed immediately. You will be pleased to know that there is no specific ethical guidance on this topic. However, achieving an adequate work/life balance does involve considering patient safety and cover issues, the ethical guidance of which has already been discussed.

Summary of question types you encounter

As you can see a lot of the model answers and the ethical guidance are taken from the GMC publication 'Good Medical Practice (2006)'. It is therefore essential what you familiarise yourself with the basic principles that the GMC has set out. Be warned however, that although the GMC has set out these guidelines, they are indeed a guide, and you need to choose the most appropriate actions provided for each question. This may involve deviating slightly from the GMC guidance if there is not a more suitable alternative provided. Try not to be too rigid in your thinking. You still need to be flexible and apply common sense to your basic knowledge. Indeed, for general practice as indeed general life, nothing is set in stone!

We hope that has given you a feel for the sort of questions you will be asked. There are a lot more issues that will become apparent as you work through the practice questions and explanations of the ethics involved will be given. Don't be disheartened. Most of the scenarios are simple common sense situations but you will encounter more complicated questions, where ethics comes into play! This book contains 70 SJTs for you to work through together with detailed explanations of the answers. The questions provided are designed to become increasingly more difficult. We will also give you some worked examples first so you can learn how to approach the questions before you start. Hopefully, by the end of working through this book you should feel confident that you will be able to answer anything that comes your way.

Chapter 3 Situational Judgement Tests Practice Questions – Worked Examples

Practice Question 1 (from the Introduction)

Upon joining a MDT team as an ST1 doctor you suspect that a senior nurse within the team is stealing prescription drugs and possibly self medicating. On closer observation you actually see the nurse steal the drugs from the cabinet at the beginning the shift prior to her conducting a ward round.

Rank in order from 1 to 5 the following actions in response to this situation. Where 1 is the most appropriate action and 5 is the least appropriate action.

A. You ignore what you have just seen. You have only been a member of the team for a matter of weeks and do not want to interfere.

B. You ask to speak with the nurse immediately with your concerns away from the ward, ensure that they do not have any contact with patients and encourage them to go home.

C. Attempt to seek the opinion of your Registrar but find that he is unavailable for the next hour.

D. You decide to raise the issue at your next appraisal to ensure that the nurse receives help.

E. You report the matter as a critical incident as per your Trusts protocol.

Suggested Approach to this Question

The best initial approach to answering a SJT is to identify the issue or dilemma at the heart of it. As stated in Chapter 2, this provides an idea on the ethical principles behind the question and also an idea on how to structure your answer. In this case the ethical dilemma is clearly an issue with the work ethic of a colleague as well as a criminal issue. Stealing prescription drugs is actually illegal and the fact that the nurse is self medicating may pose a threat to patient safety. Thus there is a potential safety issue and the matter cannot be ignored.

Option A: In view of this, the least appropriate action has to be Option A. Although you may have been a member of the team for only a few weeks, this is no excuse to ignore the situation. This is especially true for situations where patient safety may be at risk and as stated when we discussed the GMC guidance on patient safety, you must act swiftly if you feel patients may be at risk.

You are therefore left with four remaining options to rank. These four options all involve addressing the issue but with different levels of urgency and in different ways. Only one of the options (Option B) involves addressing the issue immediately and ensuring that the patients are safe, whereas the others involve dealing with the matter less urgently. If you remember the discussion in Chapter 2, you should always ensure that the patients are safeguarded first and foremost. We should rank other options that involve delaying dealing with the matter or taking preventative measures to stop it from happening again as less important.

Option B: In view of this and the fact that patients may be at risk if this nurse continues to work, the most appropriate action has to be Option B. This is the only option that deals with the situation immediately and safeguards the patient's welfare which must be the priority. Option B is the most appropriate action and should be taken first.

The three remaining options involve discussing the matter with various other people in various ways and can be ranked in view of the urgency with which they deal with the matter.

Option D: This is inappropriate on two counts. Firstly, in view of the time delay that may be involved in waiting until your next appraisal. There is no mention of when your next appraisal is and to wait until your next appraisal to mention this situation is not appropriate as you may be putting patients at risk during this time. Secondly, an appraisal is designed to discuss your progress and not to raise issues about the performance of other colleagues. It is not the correct forum within to discuss conduct issues in other colleagues.

Option E: Although reporting the matter via a critical incident form will ensure that the matter is dealt with at some point in the future, it will not deal with the matter immediately. Critical incident forms are very impersonal and as this is quite a delicate matter it may not be the most sensitive way to address the issue.

Option C: Enlisting senior help is probably a good idea as you are likely to be out of your depth here in dealing with the matter alone as a foundation doctor. As stated previously, although you do have a duty to raise issues that may be compromising patient care and safety, it is not your duty to deal with the matter alone. It is entirely appropriate to involve a senior to help in this difficult situation. However, the question states that your SpR is not available for the next hour and although that may not seem like a lot of time, you have a duty to safeguard the patients now.

In view of these comments we can now rank these remaining three options. From the discussion we can see that Option C is more appropriate than the other two options as it involves directly tackling the situation today, albeit in an hour. Although, this is not dealing with it immediately as with Option B, it will address the problem a lot sooner than completing a critical incident form or waiting until your next appraisal. It is also more appropriate to approach a senior to deal with the matter than using an incident form or your appraisal as already discussed. Option C is the 2nd most appropriate action overall.

You are now left with two rather inappropriate actions to rank. As previously stated both options involve a delay in dealing with the situation, but a critical incident form is likely to deal with the matter more swiftly that waiting until your next appraisal. Also, although it may seem quite insensitive to simply fill in an incident form about this matter, it is more appropriate than discussing the matter at your appraisal. At least critical incident forms are designed to investigate situations where patients were or potentially could have been put at risk. Your appraisal however is designed to assess your progress and development as a doctor. Option E is therefore more appropriate than Option D. This makes Option E the 3rd most appropriate option and Option D the 4th most appropriate option.

Although both Options D and E are inappropriate and do not deal with the matter immediately, they at least address the matter in some way. This is not the case with to Option A where you ignore what you have seen completely for fear of a reprisal despite putting patients at risk. Hence Option A is still the least appropriate action, as you must ignore a patient safety issue.

Suggested Answer: 1.B 2.C 3.E 4.D 5.A

Practice Question 2 (from the Introduction)

You are nearing the end of a busy shift when one of your patient's family members confronts you in the middle of the ward in a very aggressive manner regarding the standard of care their relative is receiving. You are not familiar with the patient's progress and need to leave promptly as you have an outside engagement.

Choose the 3 most appropriate actions to take out of the 7 actions below (no need to order).

    A. See if one of your colleagues who has just started their shift and has been directly involved in the treatment of the patient is available to update the relative.

    B. Request that one of the nurses addresses the situation on your behalf.

    C. Calm the relative down and assure them that you are going to personally look into their concerns.

    D. Request one of your nurse colleagues escort the relative to a consultation room to await a member of staff who can discuss their concerns.

    E. Address the situation there and then and advise the relative that they have nothing to worry about.

    F. Tell the relative that you have not been involved in the care of the patient and that they should ring the ward tomorrow morning to raise their concerns.

    G. Tell the relative that you do not work on the ward and that they should raise their concerns with someone else.

Suggested Approach to this Question

Again it is useful to think of the problem or dilemma in the question. Here you are faced with a work/life balance conflict and this question tests your professional integrity, communication and organisational skills. You are near the end of your shift, it is busy so you are likely to be tired and wanting to get home, however you are still on duty. As stated in Chapter 2, when you are faced with a SJT that is addressing a work/life balance issue you need to ensure that it does not include a patient safety issue. Although you are entitled to leave work on time you must ensure that your patients are adequately cared for before you leave. Although the relatives may simply be upset through a misunderstanding, there may actually be a problem with the standard of care their relative is receiving, and thus you do need to address the issue before you leave. Although, you may not know much about the patient's progress you do have upset relatives in front of you and you have a duty to ensure that the patient is safe. It would not be professional or courteous to ignore the relatives and it would be rude and unsafe for the patient to not take their concerns seriously.

We have therefore agreed that we cannot simply brush off this family member and leave our shift. In view of this there are two options that do exactly this and are thus inappropriate

Options F and G: Option F not only avoids addressing the issue but also involves being quite abrupt to the upset relatives. Although you may not be familiar with the patient, not even attempting to address the situation is only likely to upset the relatives further and is not professional or best practice. Also if there is indeed an issue relating to how this patient is being treated you may be causing more harm to the patient by delaying looking into the matter until tomorrow. Option G is also very similar in that you avoid handling the situation and give the relatives a rather rude response. Simply telling the relatives to speak to someone else is hardly helpful at all and you cannot simply shirk responsibility from this situation and leave your shift. Thus Options F and G are both inappropriate.

Option E: Although this option involves giving the relatives some sort of immediate response it is also not appropriate. The question clearly states that you have no idea of the patient's progress and therefore are not really in a position to tell them there and then not to worry. As previously stated there may actually be a patient safety issue that you need to deal with. Also to address the upset relatives in the middle of the ward would be insensitive and would not be protecting the patient's confidentiality and is there inappropriate for these reasons also. Therefore Option E is not really an option.

Option D: Along the same line of thought, Option D seems like a sensible idea. We have just discussed that addressing the relatives on a busy ward is not appropriate especially when we have no clue about the patient. Thus it would seem sensible to ask one of the nurses to escort the relatives to a private area where a member of staff, presumably who has been dealing with the patient will address their concerns. Although, you may not be that member of staff you are at least addressing the matter. As stated in Chapter 2, you are allowed to delegate tasks. It would seem especially appropriate in this scenario to delegate the task to someone who knows the patient. This would be more beneficial for the relatives as well as allowing you to leave on time. Thus Option D is an appropriate action.

Option B: Although you know little about this patient, asking a nurse to address the situation is even more inappropriate. Although the nurse may know if the patient is making progress in general they are unlikely to know the finer details of their medical care and thus it is not appropriate to ask them to deal with the relatives. This may also be seen as shirking responsibility and also putting another colleague in an awkward situation and although you may wish to leave on time this is not appropriate delegation. Thus Option B is not an appropriate action to take.

Option A: This option also involves asking another colleague to deal with the situation; however it is entirely different to Option B. Here you are asking another doctor, who is aware of the patient's condition, to deal with the relatives. In this way, they are more likely to be able to answer the relative's questions, and as they have just started their shift will have more time and be in a better frame of mind than you to do so. In this way you can ensure the relatives' questions are answered but it also allows you to leave on time to attend your engagement, and is an example of appropriate delegation. Thus Option A is an appropriate action to take.

Option C: By taking time out to calm the relatives down you are showing empathy and sensitivity. By assuring them you will look into the matter personally not only are you dealing with the situation but also giving yourself time to explore the facts. Although this may mean that you leave late, it is at least showing professionalism and ensuring that there is not a patient safety issue. Although we have stated before that you should try to delegate any tasks if possible to demonstrate a work/life balance, the other remaining options were inappropriate. Thus in this case you may have to accept that you need to deal with this issue and thus will be leaving later. Thus Option C is an appropriate action to take in view of the remaining options.

Suggested Answer: A. C. D

Practice Question 3

You are on call one evening as a FY2 doctor when you are bleeped to a patient undergoing convulsions following surgery and you feel the situation is well out of your clinical competency. What would you do?

Rank in order from 1 to 5 the following actions in response to this situation. Where 1 is the most appropriate action and 5 is the least appropriate action.

A. Use the situation as a learning curve to ensure that when faced with the situation again you would be able to deal with it effectively.

B. Obtain as much information as possible regarding the situation and attempt to stabilise the patient.

C. Complete a clinical incident form.

D. Plough on with addressing the situation without seeking further help as it would be a sign of weakness to admit that you do not know how to deal with the situation.

E. Request that another more senior doctor is bleeped immediately.

Suggested Approach to this Question

The dilemma here involves recognising the limits of your competency and protecting the safety of the patient. Although, you may feel embarrassed that you do not know how to handle the situation, you have a duty to protect the patient, and must take steps to do so. As this is a patient safety issue, we can use the suggested approach that we discussed in Chapter 2. Here we try to remove the risk to the patient and protect them first and foremost. Subsequently we can then take steps to investigate why the matter occurred and try to prevent it from happening, but safeguarding the patient immediately must take priority. As we have identified that the patient is at risk we cannot ignore the issue nor do anything that would further harm the patient.

Option D: In view of this the least appropriate answer is obvious. No matter how embarrassed you feel, it is not safe to plough on with the situation and risk harming the patient and making the situation worse. Thus option D must come last and is entirely inappropriate.

Conversely, the two most appropriate answers are also obvious as only two of the options (Options E and B) involve immediately making sure the patient is safe. The issue is to decide which one to rank first.

Option B: Here you try your best, within your competency limits, to stabilise the patient thus minimising the damage to the patient from the situation.

This means that you are at least trying to help the patient in some way. However, after that you are now stuck with a further plan of action as you are inexperienced in how to manage the patient further.

Option E: By asking the nurses to contact a more senior doctor immediately you are ensuring that someone trained attends to the patient as soon as possible. It makes more sense to do this first, whilst you try to find out more information about the patient. At least after you have done your best to stabilise the patient there should hopefully be someone more experienced to take over. This is safer than you trying to stabilise the patient when you know you are out of your depth before contacting someone senior. Therefore it makes more sense to rank Option E before Option B.

You are now left with two options which have nothing to do with immediately safeguarding the patient, but more with ensuring this incident does not happen again.

Option A: Here you use the experience as a learning curve, perhaps putting it in your appraisal folder. You can then address it as a learning need to ensure you are able to handle the situation, if it should arise again. This shows that you can learn from experience and that you take active steps to ensure that you keep your knowledge up to date.

Option C: This involves filling in a critical incident form which is not entirely appropriate in view of the situation. By filling in an incident form you are saying that someone or something is to blame for this situation happening. Although, you may be slightly correct in thinking this, it is actually your lack of knowledge which is the incident. It would have been different had the nurses not been able to contact a senior doctor and had no choice but to contact you instead, as this would definitely have been a critical incident. However, there is no mention of this at all and thus you cannot really blame this on anyone. Thus it is more appropriate to learn from this experience than to fill in an incident form and thus Option A ranks before Option C.

Suggested Answer: 1.E 2.B 3.A 4.C 5.D

Notes on this question

Some could argue about the prioritisation of the last two options A and C and state that an incident form is more important than using the experience as a learning curve (i.e. rank Option C before Option A). Those of you who did so may have felt that the nursing staff should have bleeped someone more senior straight away and thus a critical incident occurred. However, this is not stated in the information provided. There is no mention of any critical incident occurring and as a foundation doctor you should be able to deal with common medical emergencies. In any case the outcome of the incident form would probably be that you need to learn how to manage common medical emergencies. Thus it makes sense for you to realise this yourself and do something about your lack of knowledge immediately rather than waiting for the outcome of a critical incident form to point this out to you. Thus in the model answer Option C was less appropriate than Option A.

Some may also argue that you should attempt to obtain the information and stabilise the patient before calling the Registrar (i.e. ranked BEACD). Although you do need to stabilise the patient as your first priority it will not take much time for you to ask someone to bleep someone senior. It may have been different if the option stated that you had to call the senior yourself which would obviously distract you from addressing the patient. However, the question states that this scenario is out of your clinical competencies and although you will do what you can to stabilise the patient it is safer to request a senior is contacted sooner rather than later. However, you would have scored partial marks had you attempted to stabilise the patient and then requested for a senior to be called.

Practice Question 4

You have been in your new ST1 post for two months now and feel that one of your fellow ST1 colleagues is not really pulling their weight which is impacting on both your performance and the standard of care being provided.

Choose the 3 most appropriate actions to take out of the 7 actions below (no need to order).

A. Ring the Human Resources department and ask to discuss his performance with someone.

B. Say nothing to anyone and let one of your senior colleagues deal with the situation as his performance is not your responsibility. It is your senior's duty to realise that there is a problem and sort out the matter.

C. Ask to speak to your colleague in private regarding his performance and express your concern regarding his performance and if there is anything you can do to help.

D. Discuss your colleagues' poor performance with the rest of the team with the view of bringing it up at the next team meeting.

E. Speak to your colleague in private regarding his performance and advise them that you think it wise that they discuss the problems they are having with one of the Registrars.

F. Wait until your colleague makes a significant mistake so that you can complete a critical incident form.

G. Confide in your Registrar regarding the situation.

Suggested Approach to this Question

The dilemma here again revolves around the work ethic of a colleague. Thus we can use the approach outlined in Chapter 2 to choose the most appropriate answers. We have stated that when in this situation we need to ask ourselves if there is an issue at hand and if there could be a potential patient safety issue as this cannot be ignored. In this question there is a direct mention that your colleagues' performance is affecting the standard of care provided. Thus you have a duty to deal with the situation promptly as patient safety may be compromised if the situation is not dealt with. However, it has not happened as yet and thus it may be appropriate to try and deal with this situation tactfully before involving any outsiders.

As stated in Chapter 2, you need to be sensitive in your approach and try to deal with the matter locally and use the hierarchy of seniority appropriately. You should only involve people that are necessary to resolve the situation and should not spread rumour or gossip. Although we do have a duty to address this matter, no serious offence has occurred as yet and it may be appropriate to deal with this situation on a one-to-one basis with our colleague.

Option B: In view of the above, Option B is obviously inappropriate. Although you are not responsible for your colleagues training, you do have a responsibility to inform someone (whistle blow) if you feel patient safety may potentially be compromised. As your colleague's behaviour is impacting on the standards of care provided, if the situation is not dealt with it could potentially result in a patient safety issue. So although involving a senior would be a good idea, waiting for a senior to realise that there is a problem and handle the matter is not appropriate as you could be putting patients at risk in the meantime.

Option F: Similarly waiting until patient safety has been breached before dealing with the matter is not appropriate. The whole reason of addressing this issue is to ensure that no patient comes to harm and to deal with the matter well before this happens. Thus, to wait until a patient has been harmed before doing something about your colleague's behaviour is entirely inappropriate.

You are now left with various options of addressing your colleague's performance which involve informing different people or dealing with it on a one-to-one basis with your colleague.

Option A: As previously stated you need to deal with this matter sensitively and involve the appropriate people. HR therefore are not the best people to deal with this situation as this is not their job and this is not trying to deal with the matter as locally as possible. They are likely to inform your Consultant straight away or someone even more senior who would be more equipped to deal with the situation.

Option D: Discussing your colleague with the whole team is not appropriate and does not show any courtesy for your colleague. It is not necessary for the whole team to be involved and is unlikely to help you any more than discussing it with one member, e.g. your Registrar. Also the option states that you intend to raise the performance issues at the next team meeting. This is not appropriate in view of the fact that it is delaying dealing with the situation at hand when there could be a potential patient safety issue if left unaddressed. It is also not the most appropriate forum to discuss such a sensitive matter. Thus this option is entirely inappropriate as it is unfair to your colleague and unsafe to the patients as it involves unnecessary delay.

Option G: This option is an excellent example of how to involve the correct person in the situation. By discussing this matter with a senior who directly knows your colleague, and is involved in the team, you will be able to obtain a more senior and expert opinion. It is better to discuss this matter with your Registrar than to go to Human Resources who have probably never even met your colleague, and will probably bypass your Registrar and go straight to the Consultant on this issue. Thus Option G is an appropriate action and is more appropriate than Option A, as it involves informing a more suitable person and is fairer to your colleague. It is certainly also more appropriate than Option D where you would discuss your concerns with the entire team which would demonstrate little respect or empathy for your colleague.

Option C: Similarly, having a discussion with your colleague privately shows sensitivity and at least gives your colleague the opportunity to address the situation before informing any senior colleagues. Your colleague may be having personal problems and hence by this approach you show respect and empathy for a fellow colleague who may be having difficulties. As there has not been a patient safety breach as yet it is feasible to attempt to discuss this matter with your colleague first to see if changes could be made. Obviously the situation may have been different if a serious incident had occurred such as your colleague viewing child pornography, and it may not have been appropriate to discuss it with your colleague in this circumstance. However, in this case a simple quiet word with your colleague may suffice. Thus Option C is an appropriate action to take and is more appropriate than Options A and D.

Option E: This is similar to Option C in that you discuss your concerns with your colleague but advise him to discuss his problems with a Registrar. Although, you may feel that this is not ideal as you are now passing the responsibility onto someone else, you may also be diverting him to someone more equipped to handle the situation. Also in view of the other options e.g. speaking to human resources or discussing it with the whole team, it is a more appropriate action to take.

Suggested Answer: C. E. G

Practice Question 5

You are an ST2 doctor and feel that your Registrar is continually dumping work on you at the last minute. They do not behave like this with any of your other junior colleagues. What do you do?

Rank in order from 1 to 5 the following actions in response to this situation. Where 1 is the most appropriate action and 5 is the least appropriate action.

A. Approach your Consultant regarding the situation.
B. Ask to speak to the Registrar away from the ward regarding how you feel and how you feel the situation could be improved.
C. Confront the Registrar on the ward right now.
D. Accuse the Registrar of discrimination and that you are going to report them to the GMC.
E. Confide in one of your fellow ST2 colleagues.

Suggested Approach to this Question

The dilemma here is again one involving the work ethic of a colleague. In this situation you feel that you are being treated unfairly but you may not feel in a position as a junior to deal with the situation. However, to ignore the situation would not be conducive to a good working environment. You may become overworked and as a result not be able to provide your usual high standard of care. The situation therefore needs to be addressed, not only for your morale but for the safety of the other patients. The issue is how you address it and who you inform. As a rule when dealing with the work ethics of other colleagues, it is preferable to try and deal with the matter locally if appropriate. You should also avoid confronting colleagues in a confrontational manner and making assumptions with little evidence.

Option D: In view of the above this option immediately seems inappropriate. To accuse your Registrar of discrimination is making a wild assumption and to go to the GMC over this issue is rather drastic. This is not dealing with the matter locally as suggested by the GMC and it does not allow your colleague any chance to address the issue. It may be that the matter is a simple misunderstanding. As upset as you are it would be professional discourtesy to go behind your colleague's back and inform such a senior authority with an allegation that has no foundation at this stage. Option D is the least appropriate option as it involves assuming the worse about your colleague and going against the guidance on how we should deal with these matters and is the option that is likely to have the most adverse outcome.

Option C: Similarly confronting the Registrar on the ward is unlikely to achieve anything. You are likely to damage your relationship with the Registrar even and possibly upset patients and other staff in the process. This is not professional behaviour and it is better to calm down and think about the matter rationally instead of airing your grievances whilst you are emotional. It is however marginally better than reporting your Registrar to the GMC over this matter. Therefore although Options C and D are both inappropriate, Option C is marginally better than Option D.

You are now left with three options: two of them involve actually taking steps to address the situation (Options A and B) and one of them involves confiding in a slightly more senior colleague who is unlikely to be able to do anything about the situation themselves (Option E). It is preferable to deal with the situation at hand and thus Options A and B are likely to be more appropriate than confiding in your colleague. However, we need to analyse the remaining options before making that final decision.

Options A and B: With regards to addressing the situation you have two options; Option A where you go straight to your Consultant and Option B where you have a private talk with your Registrar to see if you can resolve the situation. Option B shows slightly more professional courtesy to your Registrar and shows that you are willing to try and improve this situation without involving seniors. Your Registrar will probably be more grateful for this approach than you going straight to the Consultant, without even discussing it with them. As stated before, the whole situation may be a misunderstanding and having a civil discussion with your Registrar may solve the entire matter and negate the need for you to even involve anyone else. Obviously, if this did not work and the situation continued you would need to involve someone else more senior. It would be better to involve the Consultant at this point as they would actually be able to do something about the situation than to involve your ST colleague who could only offer sympathy and advice. Thus Option B is the most appropriate answer and Option A is the 2nd most appropriate answer.

Option E: By confiding in one of your colleagues you may feel slightly better talking through the matter, and may receive some impartial advice, but you have not actually dealt with the situation in question which you would do through following Options A and B. This option is more beneficial than confronting your Registrar when you are upset and it may give you an opportunity to calm down and think more rationally. It is also better than making a false accusation against your Registrar and contacting the GMC. Option E is therefore the 3rd most appropriate action.

Suggested answer 1.B 2.A 3.E 4.C 5.D

Notes on this question

Some of you may have ranked going to the consultant first before talking to the Registrar (i.e. ranked ABECD). Perhaps you may have felt uncomfortable addressing the Registrar yourself and found it easier to speak to the Consultant. Although you would have been given partial marks for dealing with the situation in an appropriate and non-confrontational manner, you have gone directly to a senior without allowing your Registrar a chance to respond. Your Registrar may honestly not have realised what they were doing and it shows professional courtesy to at least discuss it with them before going to a Consultant. However, the examiners do acknowledge that some people may not feel comfortable addressing the Registrar themselves and thus you would not be marked down too harshly for approaching the Consultant first.

Also some of you may have thought that perhaps it is better to confront the Registrar than to confide with a colleague, i.e. ranked Option C in front of Option E. The reason behind this may have been that you feel it is better to actually do something about the situation directly and talking to a fellow colleague is unlikely to solve it. Although, this may be partially true, confronting your Registrar on the ward is unlikely to achieve anything and will almost certainly make matters worse. By talking to an ST colleague you may gain another perspective on the problem, and it may even calm you down so you can think more logically. Although confronting your Registrar may seem on the surface to be addressing the issue it is unlikely to have a favourable outcome or solve the problem.

Chapter 4 Situational Judgement Tests: Practice Questions

Rank in order from 1 to 5 the following actions in response to this situation. Where 1 is the most appropriate action and 5 is the least appropriate action.

A. Ask the other patients in the same bay whether they have seen the laptop or wallet and search their bedside cabinets.

B. Fill in an incident form regarding the theft.

C. Put posters up around the ward informing everyone of the theft asking all staff, patients and relatives to be vigilant about their possessions and to be on the lookout for anyone suspicious.

D. Comfort the patient who has possibly been a victim of crime and record the necessary details about the laptop and its disappearance.

E. After ascertaining the details around the alleged theft, inform the senior nurse and ask her to inform the police.

Rank in order from 1 to 5 the following actions in response to this situation. Where 1 is the most appropriate action and 5 is the least appropriate action.

A. Confront your colleague and ask him in the staff room if he is the person who stole the watch.

B. Tell the patient that you found his watch in a colleague's bag and call him into the staff room to identify the watch.

C. Have a private discussion with your colleague to try and understand what you have seen and if indeed your suspicions are correct.

D. Call the police immediately. Theft is a criminal offence.

E. Inform your Consultant of what you have seen and let him handle the matter.

Question 3

For the past month your Consultant seems constantly irritable, stressed and seems to be making a lot of simple errors. He is also turning up late to the ward rounds. Today he prescribed the wrong dose of amoxicillin on a drug chart that you were asked to change by one of the junior nurses. What do you do?

Rank in order from 1 to 5 the following actions in response to this situation. Where 1 is the most appropriate action and 5 is the least appropriate action.

A. Fill out an incident form and let the matter be investigated via that route.

B. Have a private conversation with your Consultant and let him know that you are concerned.

C. Call the GMC and discuss your concerns with them.

D. Speak to an impartial senior that you feel comfortable with and discuss your concerns.

E. Have a chat with the nurse that noticed the error and inform her about all the other errors he has made and ask for her advice.

Question 4

You are a foundation doctor in A&E and have been asked to see an alcoholic patient with a minor head injury who is obviously inebriated. He is shouting abuse at staff and is saying that he does not want to see you. What do you do?

Choose the 3 most appropriate actions to take out of the 7 actions below.

A. Ask one of your senior colleagues to see him as you do not feel comfortable seeing someone who is shouting abuse at you.

B. Review the patient with security present in case of any threat to your safety.

C. Ignore him and wait until he sobers up before you see him. He is an alcoholic and has contributed to his own injuries by becoming drunk. You should prioritise other patients.

D. Do not see him at all. He says that he does not want to see you so you should not force medical attention upon him.

E. Attempt to calm down the patient verbally, explaining why you need to see him and attend to his injuries. If he still continues to be abusive and refuses for you to examine him clearly document this in the notes.

F. Sedate the patient so that you can attend to his injury safely without any delay or interference from the patient.

G. Mention your concerns to a senior member of staff and see if a colleague can act as a chaperone whilst you examine the patient.

Question 5

You are an FY2 doctor on a general practice rotation. You have just given a child their immunisations and are writing the details of the batch number and expiry date in the notes. Whilst doing so you realise that the injection you have given is one month out of date. What do you do?

Rank in order from 1 to 5 the following actions in response to this situation. Where 1 is the most appropriate action and 5 is the least appropriate action.

A. Say nothing to the mother at the time. It is only one month out of date so everything should be okay and you do not want to worry her.

B. Explain to the mother what has happened. As you are sure that the vaccine only being one month out of date should not matter, tell the mother she does not need to worry or do anything about the matter.

C. Go and check all the vaccinations in the fridge to ensure that they are within date.

D. Explain to the mother what has happened and contact a senior for advice on what to do next.

E. Discuss the matter as a significant event at the next practice meeting.

Question 6

You are an FY2 doctor on a general practice rotation. A patient comes to you for her routine Depo-Provera injection as the nurse is off sick today. You have never given the Depo injection before but have given intramuscular injections numerous times. What do you do?

Choose the 2 most appropriate actions to take out of the 5 actions below.

A. Read the instruction leaflet and attempt to give the injection as best you can, based on your previous experience of IM injections and mention nothing of your inexperience to the patient in case she worries.

B. Explain to the patient that you have never given this injection before and rebook her with the nurse or one of the other doctors as soon as possible.

C. Explain to the patient that you have never given the Depo injection before. However, you have given several other injections so it should not be a problem. Subsequently give her the injection if she agrees for you to so.

D. Tell her that you are not trained to give the injection and advise her to go to A&E immediately to have it done.

E. Call one of your colleagues explaining the situation and see if anyone is available to come up quickly and give the injection to the patient whilst you observe for learning purposes.

Question 7

You are an FY2 doctor working in a general practice post. A young 26 year old businessman comes to you for his blood results. Although his cholesterol is entirely normal and he has no risk factors for heart disease he is demanding quite insistently that you prescribe a statin to lower his risk. What do you do?

Choose the 2 most appropriate actions to take out of the 5 actions below.

A. Prescribe a month's supply of the statin and ask him to come back and see someone else for a repeat prescription in the hope that they will be able to convince him that he does not need it any more.

B. Explore his reasons behind why he feels he needs to take a statin and try to address his health beliefs, explaining why it is not necessary and see if this changes his mind.

C. Give him the prescription of the statin as it is easier than arguing with him that he does not need it.

D. Explain to him that you do not feel it is in his best interest to have a statin but if he would like a second opinion on this he is welcome to speak to one of the other GPs.

E. Tell him simply that he does not need a statin and refuse to prescribe it.

Question 8

You are a foundation doctor on a busy medical firm. One of your colleagues has called in sick and as you were unable to secure a locum at the last minute you ended up having to do the work of two doctors that day. You have subsequently found out that the day your colleague called in sick they were actually locuming at another hospital. What do you do?

Rank in order from 1 to 5 the following actions in response to this situation. Where 1 is the most appropriate action and 5 is the least appropriate action.

A. Tell your Consultant immediately.

B. Explain to your colleague the difficult predicament they put you in and advise them that if this happens again you feel you have no option but to involve your seniors.

C. Do nothing. No harm was caused.

D. Contact medical personnel and inform them of the lie.

E. Bring it up in your next appraisal with your educational supervisor.

Question 9

One of your elderly patients recently brought you a box of chocolates for looking after her when she was quite unwell. You graciously accepted the gift. Since then during her last two visits she has brought you chocolates both times. She now attends for her routine appointment again with chocolates. What do you do?

Choose the 3 most appropriate actions to take out of the 7 actions below.

A. Accept the chocolates graciously. It is a simple gift that was well deserved so you do not feel too concerned.
B. Tell her that she should not bring you any more gifts in case anyone gets suspicious.
C. Try to enquire politely the reasons behind the continuation of her giving you gifts, and suggest that as it was the practice as a team that contributed to her recovery, you will share the chocolates with the practice staff.
D. Accept the chocolates but secretly share them out with the rest of the practice and continue to do this whenever the patient comes in with chocolates.
E. Explain to her that there is no need to keep on giving you gifts as you will always provide her with the best care you can regardless. Politely refuse the chocolates. If she insists accept the chocolates.
F. Explain to her that there is no need to keep on giving you gifts as you will always provide her with the best care you can regardless. If she insists accept the gift but write a business like letter of thanks from the practice to acknowledge the gift.
G. Accept the chocolates but give them to the local residential home to share out amongst the residents.

Question 10

An elderly patient brings you some vegetables from his allotment to say thank you for looking after him when he was unwell on your ward. What do you do?

Choose the 3 most appropriate actions to take out of the 7 actions below.

A. Graciously accept the gift.
B. Decline the gift telling him it would not be appropriate for you to accept it as it may be viewed as suspicious.
C. Advise him that there was no need to bring you a gift as his recovery was gift enough.
D. Advise him that as his care was a team effort you will share the vegetables out with the other staff.

E. Tell him that you are not going to accept the gift as you do not like vegetables.

F. Accept the gift and ask him if he can bring you some more vegetables next week.

G. Tell him that you will have to ask your Consultant if it would be appropriate to accept the gift.

Question 11

It is your birthday and you have a big party planned for which you need to arrive on time. In view of this you have asked the doctor covering the night shift to come in half an hour early for handover so that you could leave on time. They are ten minutes late already and you are worried that you will not be able to leave on time. What do you do?

Choose the 3 most appropriate actions to take out of the 7 actions below.

A. Call them to see how far away they are and remind them that they need to hurry up as you need to leave and you are not happy that they are late.

B. Wait patiently until they arrive. Their shift doesn't technically start for another 20 minutes so you cannot do much else until they come.

C. Wait until they arrive then rush handover so you can get out on time.

D. Call your party friends to tell them that you may be slightly late but will update them further when you know more.

E. Call your colleague to see how far away they are and ask them if it is all right if you give a detailed handover to the night Registrar, who is here already. You will wait until they arrive but leave it to the Registrar to hand over to them when they arrive so you can leave on time.

F. Wait another ten minutes and then leave if they are not there, passing your handover list to one of the nursing staff in the process.

G. Ask your Registrar to call your colleague and find out where they are as they are late and you are not happy.

Question 12

You are the on call doctor and have to cover all the wards after 5pm. Thus you have to look after patients that may not necessarily be yours. A nurse bleeps you to ask you to speak to a patient's relatives who are very angry that their relative has not been moved to the local residential home and is still on the ward despite being told she would be moved a week ago. You have never seen this patient and have no clue about any details pertaining to them since their admission. What do you do?

Rank in order from 1 to 5 the following actions in response to this situation. Where 1 is the most appropriate action and 5 is the least appropriate action.

A. Explain politely to the relatives that it may be best if they speak tomorrow to the regular team looking after the patient as you do not normally look after the patient.

B. Ask the nurse on the ward to speak to the relatives as she is likely to know more about the patient's current situation.

C. Explain to the relatives that you are happy to speak to them and try to help. However you may not be able to answer all their questions as you are not on the team looking after the patient and can only go by what has been written in the notes.

D. Inform the relatives from the outset that if they wish to make a complaint they should contact the Patient Advisory and Liaison Service as you are not in a position to answer their questions.

E. Call the Consultant that is responsible for the patient explaining that the relatives are angry and unhappy and ask him to help you answer their questions as to why the patient has not been moved.

Question 13

A routine chest x-ray you requested for a well 54 year old patient with a cough comes back showing a 'shadow' on the lung. The radiologist comments that he cannot ascertain the nature of the shadow so suggests a referral to the chest clinic. Your patient asks you 'is it cancer doctor'? What do you do?

Choose the 2 most appropriate actions to take out of the 5 actions below.

A. Explain sensitively that the shadowing could possibly represent cancer but you are referring her for more tests to find out for certain.
B. Tell her that it is likely to be cancer so she can be prepared.
C. Suggest that perhaps she comes back with a relative or good friend before you discuss the answer to that question.
D. Explain to the patient that although the shadowing could represent cancer it could also represent other possibilities, for example old scarring or infection.
E. Tell her that it is better for the chest clinic to answer this question after their tests as you are not sure at this point in time and therefore not in a position to comment.

Question 14

You are an FY2 doctor on call with a locum Registrar. You are concerned that he is making inappropriate diagnoses and management decisions. What do you do?

Rank in order from 1 to 5 the following actions in response to this situation. Where 1 is the most appropriate action and 5 is the least appropriate action.

A. Nothing. He is a Registrar so knows more than you. You have probably misinterpreted the situation.
B. Contact the Consultant on call immediately and inform him of your concerns.
C. Contact medical staffing and ask them to find a replacement.
D. Challenge his decisions in front of the patients and tell him how you feel the situation should be managed differently and why.
E. Leave your shift as you are not happy to continue to work with this doctor especially as you may be held accountable for his bad decisions.

Question 15

During a night shift you are called to see an elderly dehydrated patient whose blood pressure has dropped. You prescribe IV fluids and tell the nurse looking after the patient that they should be started immediately. However, when you come to review the patient 30 minutes later the fluids have still have not been put up and his blood pressure is even lower. What do you do?

Rank in order from 1 to 5 the following actions in response to this situation. Where 1 is the most appropriate action and 5 is the least appropriate action.

A. Put the IV fluids up yourself although you are unsure of how to do this correctly as you have never done this before.
B. Fill in a critical incident form.
C. Ask one of the nurses immediately to put up the IV fluids and ensure it is done.
D. Confront in the middle of the ward the nurse who you had told to put up the fluids to enquire why it had not been done.
E. Call your Registrar and inform him of the situation and ask for further advice.

Question 16

You are a foundation doctor working in general practice. You were asked to sign a prescription by reception for Zoladex injections for a patient. You were told by the receptionist that the patient has been getting these regularly as he has prostate cancer and signed it quickly as you were busy. After attending to the nurse for his injection you find a letter from his Consultant informing you they had stopped the Zoladex one month ago. The letter was present in the notes at the time you signed the prescription. What do you do?

Choose the 3 most appropriate actions to take out of the 7 actions below.

A. Inform the nurse that she should not have given the injection when there was a letter in his notes clearly stating that the Zoladex had been stopped.
B. Organise a practice meeting to discuss the incident and perform a significant event analysis, keeping it anonymous, to see how this matter could be prevented in the future.
C. Inform the receptionists that it is unsafe for them to ask you to sign prescriptions quickly and that they should not do this moving forward to avoid any future errors.
D. Call the patient and inform him about the mistake. Reassure him that he will come to no long term harm and that you are looking into the matter so that it does not happen again.

E. Enquire as to who had seen the original letter and filed it and ask them why they did not document clearly in his notes or medications that the Zoladex was to be stopped.

F. Discuss the matter with your trainer. Inform them of the incident and discuss ways you can learn from this event. Discuss your feelings around the incident and reflect upon it.

G. Ask one of your fellow foundation doctor colleagues for advice.

Question 17

You are nearing the end of a very tedious shift when you realise that medication you administered to your last patient was incorrect resulting in a mild overdose. What do you do?

Choose the 3 most appropriate actions to take out of the 7 actions below.

A. Consult a senior colleague regarding how to proceed as this is the first time that you have made an error of this type.

B. Inform the patient and record the event in their patient notes.

C. Complete a critical incident form.

D. Review the medication guidelines and possible side effects that could arise from a mild overdose.

E. Inform the ward nurse that everything is fine.

F. Inform your Consultant the following day.

G. Bring up the error in your next ward meeting.

Question 18

You need to give your Consultant some notes and are on your way to his office. As you walk into your Consultant's office you see him putting a bottle of alcohol into his office drawer. What do you do?

Rank in order from 1 to 5 the following actions in response to this situation. Where 1 is the most appropriate action and 5 is the least appropriate action.

A. Report the matter to the GMC.

B. Nothing. It is probably a gift from one of the patient's and there is no need to take this further.

C. Ask your Consultant politely about the bottle of alcohol to see if he can offer a reasonable explanation.

D. Ask his secretary if she has noticed anything strange about your Consultant and whether she has caught him drinking on the job.

E. Tell your Consultant that in view of what you saw you are slightly worried about him and advise him to see his GP.

Question 19

The senior nurse on the ward comes to you and asks you to speak to one of your fellow junior colleagues about her dress code. She has noted that she is wearing a short skirt that she feels is inappropriate and asks you to discuss this matter with her. What do you do?

Choose the 3 most appropriate actions to take out of the 7 actions below.

A. Politely mention to your colleague that perhaps she should change her attire but do not tell her why or what has been said.

B. Ask the nurse to speak to the person in question herself or to discuss it with your Registrar as you do not feel comfortable in addressing this situation.

C. Discuss the matter informally and sensitively with your colleague informing her of what has been said by the senior nurse.

D. Tell the nurse you will speak to her but secretly do nothing. You see nothing wrong with the way she is dressed and it is not your job to tell her about this.

E. Inform medical personnel of the issue and ask them to deal with it.

F. Inform your Registrar about the complaint raised and ask them to deal with the matter.

G. Ask your fellow colleagues in the mess for advice on whether you should inform her or not.

Question 20

A single mother comes to you worried about her two year old son who has a common cold with a slight temperature and been suffering a runny nose for the past day. She is very stressed as she has three other children to look after. You advise her that this is a viral illness and that it will settle in a few days and that she should simply use paracetamol suspension. However she refuses to listen to this and is demanding antibiotics as she has no time for a sick child. What do you do?

Choose the 2 most appropriate actions to take out of the 5 actions below.

A. Give her the antibiotics as she is upset and it is easier than arguing with her.

B. Sympathise with her that it must be stressful dealing with an ill child but that antibiotics are unlikely to help and may have side effects. Explain again why you feel it is not in his best interests to have them.

C. Tell her once again that you refuse to prescribe them as antibiotics are not necessary and you will not argue about it.

D. Offer her a delayed prescription of antibiotics that she can use if her son continues to have a fever and be unwell, but advise her to hold off for now, as things are likely to improve by themselves.

E. Ask her to go and rebook to see another one of your colleagues if she is unhappy with your advice.

Question 21

You have been asked to conduct an audit for the department. You are required to show your raw data to your supervisor tomorrow afternoon. You have to look through ten more patient notes in order to complete your data but it is 3am and you are exhausted and falling asleep. The notes are quite large and it will take you at least an hour to look through the notes properly. You also have to be at work tomorrow for your shift which starts at 9am. What do you do?

Choose the 2 most appropriate actions to take out of the 5 actions below.

A. Drink some coffee and try to stay up and complete the data.

B. Make up the data for the last ten patients. As it is only ten patients it should not really make that much of a difference.

C. Go to bed and admit to your supervisor that you were unable to complete the data. However, you only have ten more patient's notes to look through so you should have the data ready by the following day.

D. Cancel your meeting with your supervisor tomorrow making up an excuse as to why you are unable to make it.

E. Go to bed and try to complete as much as the data that you can in your lunch break tomorrow.

Question 22

You work on a busy ward and share your workload with another junior doctor. You have just commenced this job but ever since you have started your colleague leaves her shift 30 minutes early. What do you do?

Rank in order from 1 to 5 the following actions in response to this situation. Where 1 is the most appropriate action and 5 is the least appropriate action.

A. Do nothing. It is only 30 minutes and if you're honest nothing really happens in the last 30 minutes of your shift.

B. Go straight to your Consultant and inform him of your colleague leaving early persistently.

C. Speak to some of your colleague's friends and the staff on the ward to see if they are aware of any problems that your colleague may be having.

D. Confront your colleague and inform them that if she does not start to pull her weight you will have to approach your seniors.

E. Approach your colleague discretely and have an informal chat with her, expressing your concerns sensitively, and try to find out the reasons behind your colleague leaving early.

Question 23

Whilst at a leaving party for one of the nurses, you overhear some of the other nurses gossiping about how they fancy one of the new hospital porters. What do you do?

Rank in order from 1 to 5 the following actions in response to this situation. Where 1 is the most appropriate action and 5 is the least appropriate action.

A. Choose a tactful time after the party to inform the nurses that their behaviour was not professional and could be interpreted wrongly by others.

B. Discuss the issue with your Consultant and ask him to address the issue.
C. Confront the nurses there and then and ask them to keep their voices down as their conversation is not professional.
D. Do nothing.
E. Inform one of the senior nurses about their behaviour and ask them to speak to the nurses on your behalf.

Question 24

A mature and intelligent 14 year old patient comes to see you with her mother. Her mother is concerned as she says that she is quite moody lately and will not tell her what is wrong. After speaking to the patient alone you discover that she has just broken up with her boyfriend and that is why she is feeling a bit down. She asks you not to tell her mother about her having a boyfriend. What do you do?

Rank in order from 1 to 4 the following actions in response to this situation. Where 1 is the most appropriate action and 4 is the least appropriate action.

A. Tell her mother about her boyfriend as she is only 14 and as she is upset and down you cannot be sure that her boyfriend did not harm her in any way.
B. Explain to the mother that you cannot reveal what you and her daughter have discussed due to confidentiality reasons.
C. Reassure the patient that what has been said will remain confidential but suggest she talks to her mother as she is obviously very concerned.
D. Inform social services of this matter.

Question 25

A 30 year old patient confides in you that she and her partner, who is also your patient, are having problems. She tells you that about a month ago he slapped her and hit one of their children. He is becoming more aggressive and she fears he will hit her again. She does not wish to contact the police and asks you not to say anything to anyone as she wishes to try and work at the marriage. What do you do?

Choose the 2 most appropriate actions to take out of the 5 actions below.

A. Respect her wishes and say nothing.
B. Call the police straight away.
C. Contact social services whether she consents or not for you to do so.
D. Call her partner informing him that you are aware of his violence and that he should book an appointment to see you.
E. Give her the details of local women's refuges and domestic violence help lines should she change her mind about her current situation.

Question 26

A 22 year old patient comes to you with some old bruises on her arms. She tells you that she walked into a door but on further questioning she reveals to you that she acquired them during an argument with her partner. She does not wish to take this matter any further. What do you do?

Rank in order from 1 to 5 the following actions in response to this situation. Where 1 is the most appropriate action and 5 is the least appropriate action.

A. Nothing. She does not wish to take this any further so you close the matter and move on.
B. Call the police. She has been assaulted and this is an offence.
C. Document everything clearly, including her injuries in case she changes her mind and this goes to court.
D. Advise her that she is well within her right to not take this matter further but advise her of her options, sources of support and the procedures should she change her mind.
E. Take this matter up with her partner as he is also your patient and tell him that his behaviour is unacceptable.

Question 27

You have just completed a night shift and are waiting to hand over to your day colleague before you can go home to rest. You have to come back later this evening to do another night shift and are keen to get some sleep. Your day colleague however is already 45 minutes late and you have no idea what has happened to him. What do you do?

Rank in order from 1 to 5 the following actions in response to this situation. Where 1 is the most appropriate action and 5 is the least appropriate action.

A. Hand over to the Consultant present with you on the post-take ward round and go home.

B. Leave a detailed handover list in the staff room for the day doctor and go home. Tell the rest of the team to let your colleague or his cover know that the list is there.

C. Call your colleague to see what the delay is and if he doesn't answer call medical staffing to see if he has called in sick.

D. Hand over to the Registrar on for the day and leave your bleep with him.

E. Offer to stay and help out either until your colleague arrives or a suitable replacement arrives even if you need to cover the entire day shift.

Question 28

You have just finished your shift and have left the hospital some 30 minutes ago. You are rushing as you are late for an important family dinner. Whilst driving you remember that you have forgotten to write up some routine eight hourly maintenance IV fluids for a patient. You try to call the on call FY2 doctor but they are not answering. What do you do?

Rank in order from 1 to 5 the following actions in response to this situation. Where 1 is the most appropriate action and 5 is the least appropriate action.

A. Go to your dinner and try to call again later in the evening.

B. Go back to the hospital to write up the fluids even if it makes you late for dinner.

C. Call the SHO to ask them to write up the fluids for you as you had forgotten and you cannot contact the FY2 doctor.

D. Call your ward and inform the senior nurse that you had forgotten to write up the fluids and if they could please bleep the on call doctor as you have not been able to get through.

E. Nothing. The nurses will realise that there are no further fluids and will bleep the on call doctor themselves.

Question 29

A mother brings her eight year old son into A&E. He is having a severe asthma attack and is extremely unwell. His mother tells you that he ran out of inhalers last month and she has not had a chance to get any more from the GP. She also tells you that his lips went blue last night and he stopped breathing but she did not call an ambulance. When you ask why she did not seek medical attention she tells you she is a single mother and didn't want to have to wake up her other children. What do you do?

Rank in order from 1 to 5 the following actions in response to this situation. Where 1 is the most appropriate action and 5 is the least appropriate action.

A. Reprimand her and point out that in addition to ensuring he had his inhalers she should have called an ambulance last night regardless of her other children.

B. Nothing. You should not judge her as you have no idea what her life is like or the pressures she is under.

C. Call social services straight away.

D. Discuss the matter with the on call paediatrician and ask for further advice.

E. Treat the child for his asthma but write a letter to his GP explaining your concerns and ask him to investigate this further.

Question 30

You are a foundation doctor on a general practice rotation. One of the medical students attached to your practice confides in you that he is very upset about his teaching on this rotation. He has exams approaching and is very anxious as he has not seen many patients with clinical signs. He has a clinical OSCE coming up and therefore needs this experience to pass his exam. What do you do?

Choose the 3 most appropriate actions to take out of the 7 actions below.

A. Tell him not to worry he is likely to pass anyway.

B. Advise him to discuss this matter with his medical school after his attachment so that they can address this matter for the future.

C. Suggest that perhaps he discuss his concerns with the GP responsible for his training so that they can arrange for him to see more patients.

D. Have a friendly chat with all the doctors in the practice asking them to please call the medical student in if they see any patients with good clinical signs as he is getting slightly worried with exams coming up.

E. Advise him to contact his medical school straight away as it is unacceptable that he is not receiving adequate teaching and he should inform them about the lack of teaching from this practice.

F. Offer to help him out with his exam revision as you have recently sat your finals. Reassure him that you will call him in if you see any patients with clinical signs and that he can come to you for any help he may need.

G. Have a word with his trainer telling him that the medical student is not happy at all as he is not getting adequate teaching and you feel something needs to be done about this immediately.

Question 31

You are a foundation doctor on a busy medical firm. It is the night after the mess party and one of your junior colleagues arrives on the ward looking very hung over and still smelling of alcohol. What do you do?

Choose the 3 most appropriate actions to take out of the 7 actions below.

A. Inform your Consultant immediately.

B. Take your colleague aside and explain to him that as he is hung over and smells of alcohol, you think it is best for him to go home for a while and that he should inform medical staffing that he is not able to stay.

C. Do nothing. Being hung over does not mean that you are unsafe to see patients.

D. Advise your colleague sensitively that perhaps next time he should stop drinking a little earlier in the evening in order to still be fit for his shift the next day.

E. Advise your colleague that he goes to see his GP to discuss his drinking habits.

F. Ask your colleague to hand over any immediate jobs to you until cover arrives. He should not be allowed to do any ward jobs in that state.

G. Inform the GMC.

Question 32

One of the ward medical nursing staff confides in you that her husband of ten years has recently been diagnosed with HIV. She is naturally very worried but is too scared to get tested. She asks you to keep this information to yourself. What do you do?

Choose the 3 most appropriate actions to take out of the 7 actions below.

A. Do nothing. It is her partner who is HIV-positive and not her. There is no need to address this issue any further.

B. Inform your occupational health department.

C. Do nothing as she is not involved in any exposure prone procedures so her HIV status does not matter.

D. Advise her for her own health if nothing else she should get tested. At least then if she does test positive she would be able to receive treatment.

E. Speak to one of your senior colleagues for advice, leaving the nurse anonymous.

F. Tell her that as she is well she is probably HIV-negative so there is no need to worry.

G. Encourage her to go and see her GP to discuss this matter and her concerns further.

Question 33

You are just about to leave for the day and stumble upon one of your junior colleagues sitting on the ward with their own laptop viewing what appears to be child pornography. What do you do?

Rank in order from 1 to 5 the following actions in response to this situation. Where 1 is the most appropriate action and 5 is the least appropriate action.

A. Confront your colleague there and then about what you have seen.

B. Inform your Consultant of what you saw.

C. Make a joke out of the situation and forget about it. It's probably nothing.

D. Report the matter to the police as child pornography is illegal.

E. Contact the Clinical Director of the hospital.

Question 34

A patient complains to you that they saw one of your colleagues reading adult pornography in the canteen. On further investigation you find out that the pornography she was referring to was Page 3 of The Sun newspaper. What do you do?

Choose the 3 most appropriate actions to take out of the 7 actions below.

A. Tell the patient that Page 3 does not really count as adult pornography and that they should not be so ridiculous.
B. Go to a senior immediately. This constitutes adult pornography and is a serious matter.
C. Do nothing.
D. Contact the GMC.
E. Apologise to the patient for what she has seen and advise her that you will discuss the matter with your colleague.
F. Contact the police.
G. Have a private conversation with your colleague regarding the complaint the patient has made and suggest that although this situation may be entirely innocent, perhaps he should apologise to the patient to ensure the matter does not escalate.

Question 35

You are a foundation doctor on a general practice post. A patient comes to see you looking slightly pale and unwell. He is Polish and speaks no English at all, however is pointing to his chest and can just about tell you that he has pain there. You cannot seem to understand anything else he is saying. What do you do?

Choose the 2 most appropriate actions to take out of the 5 actions below.

A. Do an ECG immediately and abandon trying to take a history.
B. Try to obtain some sort of history out of him with the use of pictures and diagrams no matter how long it takes to figure out what is going on.
C. Call an ambulance explaining that he speaks no English at all so you were unable to obtain a history
D. Ask the patient to rebook with a Polish interpreter.
E. Tell the patient to go straight to A&E

Question 36

You are a foundation doctor currently working in an A&E post. One of your patients presents recurrently with chest pain which has always been found to be of non-cardiac origin. You suspect that the underlying problem is psychosocial but they are demanding that you ask one of the cardiology doctors to review them. What do you do?

Rank in order from 1 to 5 the following actions in response to this situation. Where 1 is the most appropriate action and 5 is the least appropriate action.

A. Explain that it may be more appropriate to be seen as an outpatient and suggest that they ask their GP to refer them as an outpatient.

B. Attempt to explain to them that the tests they have had have excluded any heart problem and try to reassure them that there is unlikely to be anything wrong with their heart.

C. Ask the on call psychiatrist to come and see the patient as you are sure there is some underlying psychosocial problem.

D. Ask one of your senior colleagues to come and speak to the patient to reassure them that you have excluded any pathology with their heart.

E. Bleep the on call doctor and refer the patient to them as a suspected acute coronary syndrome, even though you have excluded any medical cause of the chest pain.

Question 37

You are a FY2 doctor on a GP rotation. One of your patients, is also a doctor, and comes to you to admit he has been drinking a lot of late, as he is having marital problems. He feels it is now getting out of control. He asks you to keep this information to yourself as he is scared he will lose his job. What do you do?

Choose the 3 most appropriate actions to take out of the 7 actions below.

A. Contact the GMC. He is a danger to patients.

B. Assess the situation. If his drinking seems under control, and he is not posing any immediate danger to patients, advise him on local counselling services for doctors and perhaps given him a medical certificate to have some time off work until he gets the matter sorted.

C. Ask him to come back and see one of the senior partners as you feel slightly out of your depth in dealing with this situation.

D. Keep the information to yourself, and do nothing. Ask him to come back if he feels he is a danger to patients.

E. Ask him if he would mind if you discuss his situation with one of the senior partners as you are unsure as to how to handle the situation.

F. Inform him that you will support him in any way you can. However, if he continues to work or his situation deteriorates you may have to break confidentiality and inform his employer.

G. Call his wife to see if she can help in the matter and whether she would consider going to marriage counselling with him.

Question 38

You are an FY2 doctor on a general practice rotation. A competent 88 year old lady has recently been diagnosed with iron deficiency anaemia. When you explain to her the possible causes she tells you that she does not want any investigations to find out the cause. What do you do?

Choose the 3 most appropriate actions to take out of the 7 actions below.

A. Explain to her that it is in her best interests to have it investigated and refer her for a colonoscopy and gastroscopy regardless of how she feels.

B. Explain to her that as she is declining any investigations you will have no choice but to contact her next of kin to ask them for their permission to investigate this further.

C. Explore her reasons for not wanting to have any further investigations and allay any concerns if possible.

D. Explain to her the advantages and disadvantages of having the investigations versus not having any but ultimately leave the decision down to her.

E. Mention the situation to her daughter, who is also a patient, and if her daughter agrees that she needs to be investigated then refer her on.

F. Suggest she discusses the matter with her family and next of kin and come back to you with her final decision. If she still declines accept her wishes.

G. Agree that as she is 88 there is no point in investigating her anyway as they are unlikely to do anything about it should anything sinister be found.

Question 39

You are an FY2 doctor on a medical rotation. You are bleeped on a night shift at 5am to ask you attend the ward as a demented patient is wandering the ward and won't stay in their bed. You arrive on the ward and the patient is walking around the ward quietly but all the other patients are sleeping and are undisturbed. The nurse in charge asks you to sedate the patient as they are unable to cope with the patient. What do you do?

Rank in order from 1 to 5 the following actions in response to this situation. Where 1 is the most appropriate action and 5 is the least appropriate action.

A. Sedate the patient as he is causing a bother to the nursing staff and may affect their ability to care for the other patients.

B. Try to encourage the patient to go back to bed and remain on the ward for a while if necessary until the patient settles.

C. Ask the nursing staff to bleep the Registrar to ask them to sedate the patient as you are not comfortable with doing it yourself.

D. Explain to the nursing staff that you do not feel comfortable sedating the patient, although you appreciate the inconvenience to them. You will discuss the matter with the Consultant on the ward round tomorrow to ensure that something is done about it.

E. Reprimand the nursing staff informing them that they should be used to dealing with demented patients and it is not acceptable to sedate a patient just because they cannot cope with the situation and you therefore refuse to sedate the patient.

Question 40

There is five minutes to go until you finish your day shift. You have made plans with friends that evening and are keen to leave on time having finished late most days this week. Your bleep suddenly goes off just as you have left the ward. You check your bleep and it is your ward that is bleeping you. What do you do?

Choose the 3 most appropriate actions to take out of the 7 actions below.

A. Ignore the bleep. There is only five minutes to go until you are officially off duty and if it's that important they will bleep the on call doctor.

B. Answer the bleep and deal with the matter even if it means staying back late. Your friends will have to wait.

C. Answer the bleep, and if it is not urgent, explain that you are finishing your shift and if they could please bleep the on call doctor.

D. Answer the bleep to find out the problem and hand over to the on call doctor yourself, explaining that you have just been bleeped but you would like to be able to leave on time.

E. Ask a colleague who is still doing some duties on their ward to answer the bleep for you.

F. Ask one of the nurses to answer the bleep for you and explain that you have already left for the day.

G. Go back to the ward to see what the problem is. If it is not urgent ask the nurse to bleep the on call doctor as you would like to be able to leave on time.

Question 41

You are the on call surgical foundation doctor on a busy shift and have had several referrals and it is not even lunchtime. It is your first day on the attachment. The Registrar accepts all GP referrals, however as he is busy in theatre with an emergency he gives you his bleep to hold and answer. A GP bleeps him, wanting some advice on a complex patient with abdominal pain who he thinks may need admission. What do you do?

Rank in order from 1 to 5 the following actions in response to this situation. Where 1 is the most appropriate action and 5 is the least appropriate action.

A. Advise him as best you can based on your current, but insufficient surgical knowledge.

B. Go and relay the information the GP has given you to the Registrar in theatre and see whether he will accept the referral or if he has any advice for the GP. Tell the GP you will ring him back with the Registrar's advice.

C. Explain to the GP that you cannot accept referrals and advise him to contact one of the other Registrars for advice as the on call Registrar is in theatre. If he cannot get through to anyone else then he may ring you back.

D. Accept the referral, and let the Registrar review the patient later, explaining to him why you accepted the referral.

E. Explain to the GP that you cannot accept referrals and thus he will need to try and contact the Registrar at a later time as he is busy with an emergency right now.

Question 42

A patient has come to see you with regard to her back pain. She spends most of the consultation however telling you how one of your colleagues is useless, does not listen to her and refuses to refer her for a scan. What do you do?

Rank in order from 1 to 5 the following actions in response to this situation. Where 1 is the most appropriate action and 5 is the least appropriate action.

   A. Advise her that if she has an issue with one of your colleagues it is best she discusses this matter with him as you do not feel you are in a position to comment.
   B. Advise her that if she is truly unhappy with the care she has been given by your colleague she is free to make a complaint and advise her of the complaints procedure.
   C. Agree with the patient that she has been mismanaged by your colleague and ensure her that you will not do the same.
   D. Listen to her patiently without commenting on your colleague's behaviour. Empathise with her concerns and see what her response is. If she is still very unhappy enquire as to whether she wishes to make a formal complaint.
   E. Call a practice meeting to discuss this issue and your colleague's behaviour.

Question 43

You are currently in a post in Obstetrics and Gynaecology and are in theatre for the morning session. The Registrar has been called to deal with an emergency on the ward and the Consultant asks you to assist in theatre with the next case whilst he is away. The next case is a termination of pregnancy which you are against due to religious beliefs. What do you do next?

Rank in order from 1 to 4 the following actions in response to this situation. Where 1 is the most appropriate action and 4 is the least appropriate action.

A. Inform the Consultant that you are unable to assist as it is against your religious beliefs and ask him to find someone else as you are leaving theatre.

B. Do not assist in the procedure and resign from your job today. You are not happy to perform in any procedures that are against your religious beliefs.

C. Assist in the procedure without question as you should not let your religious beliefs affect patient care.

D. Bleep one of your colleagues to see if they can assist in the procedure until the Registrar returns, but if they are unavailable assist until the Registrar returns.

Question 44

One of your very wealthy elderly patients comes to see you after you recently referred her to a surgeon with suspected bowel cancer. Her tumour was resected, as it was caught early, and she was given the all clear. She mentions to you that she would like to make you a beneficiary in her will in view of the care you provided. What do you do?

Rank in order from 1 to 5 the following actions in response to this situation. Where 1 is the most appropriate action and 5 is the least appropriate action.

A. Advise her that as it was the surgeons who resected the tumour and perhaps she should discuss making them a beneficiary of her will, not yourself.

B. Advise her that you are flattered by her offer but that you cannot accept her offer due to professional regulations and guidance by the GMC.

C. Accept the offer graciously; after all it was you who diagnosed the cancer early, but encourage her to inform her family of her decision.

D. Decline the offer politely but suggest she makes a smaller donation to the practice instead as a token of her gratitude.

E. Accept the offer graciously; after all it was you who diagnosed the cancer early, but ask her not to inform her family of her decision in case they disagree.

Question 45

You are an FY2 doctor on a general practice post. Several of your patients have complained about the nursing standards at your local hospital. Today yet another patient complains about the standard of nursing they received whilst as an inpatient. What do you do?

Choose the 3 most appropriate actions to take out of the 7 actions below.

A. Contact the Nursing and Midwifery Council and raise your concerns to them.

B. Advise them to contact the local PALS service immediately at the hospital to raise their concerns and give them the contact details.

C. Wait until the next practice meeting, and then discuss the matter with the partners at the practice.

D. Advise the patient to contact the local media to raise their concerns.

E. Do nothing. You cannot verify if their complaints are justified so you are not in a position to do anything.

F. Have an informal talk with the Director of Nursing at the hospital mentioning the complaints you have received.

G. Put your concerns in writing to the Clinical Director of the hospital expressing what your concerns are.

Question 46

A 32 year old patient comes to you requesting a termination. She is married and was not using any contraception yet does not wish to continue with the pregnancy. You are unhappy to refer her yourself for termination as it is not only against your religious beliefs but you do not feel she has genuine reasons to terminate. What do you do?

Rank in order from 1 to 4 the following actions in response to this situation. Where 1 is the most appropriate action and 4 is the least appropriate action.

A. Tell her to go private as she got herself into this predicament by not using any contraception and therefore you do not feel comfortable referring her for a termination as you feel it is not necessary.

B. Tell her you would not feel comfortable referring her for termination due to your religious beliefs, but will ask another doctor in the practice to see her who does not share your views.

C. Tell her you would not feel comfortable referring her as it is against your religious beliefs but give her the numbers of local family planning clinics who will be able to refer her.

D. Tell her than you cannot refer her for termination as you feel she does not have a reason to terminate this pregnancy. Explain she should have been using contraception if she did not want to become pregnant. Advise her to see one of your other colleagues in the surgery.

Question 47

A new patient has just registered with your surgery. It is the Friday before a bank holiday weekend and they are asking the reception for a repeat prescription for a month's supply of temazepam 20mgs tablets. They have asked you if it is okay to issue a prescription for the patient. What do you do?

Choose the 3 most appropriate actions to take out of the 7 actions below.

A. Do not give the prescription as there are no notes, and ask the patient to book an appointment on the Tuesday after the bank holiday weekend to discuss this matter with you personally.

B. Ask the patient to book an appointment with you as soon as she can, but give her 14 days supply so she does not run out in the meantime, just in case she cannot get an appointment.

C. Contact the patient's GP to get her repeat prescription information. If you confirm she is on repeat temazepam 20mgs give her the 28 days' supply.

D. Give the patient a few tablets to last the bank holiday weekend but ask her to come in on the Tuesday to discuss the matter with you. Advise her that she will not get any more medication until she has done so.

E. Tell the patient to go to A&E to get the prescription as you are reluctant to give it as she has no notes.

F. Give the patient enough for today but tell the patient to call the out of hours GP on the weekend to get more.

G. Contact the patient's GP to get her repeat prescription information. If you confirm she is on repeat temazepam, still only give her a very small supply and ask her to come and see you next week.

Question 48

You have informed one of your patients who is a bus driver that he should stop driving due to his medical condition. You informed him clearly that he should inform the DVLA himself and the reasons for this. Whilst boarding a busy bus the following weekend, you realise that your patient is the bus driver. What do you do?

Rank in order from 1 to 4 the following actions in response to this situation. Where 1 is the most appropriate action and 4 is the least appropriate action.

A. Inform him quietly there and then on the bus that he should not be driving as it is unsafe for him to do so.

B. Say nothing at the time but then call the patient to ask him to book an appointment to see you to discuss the matter.

C. Contact the bus depot and inform them of the fact that he should not be driving and that they need to fire him from his job.

D. Call the patient after the incident to inform him that if he does not stop driving you will have no option but to contact the DVLA.

Question 49

You have had concerns about your Registrar who seems to be making a lot of clinical errors, many of which have put patients at risk. You have discussed it with your Consultant but it is not apparent that he has done anything about the situation. Today your Registrar misdiagnosed a patient and this resulted in the patient becoming quite unwell. Your Consultant again has just shrugged off the incident. What do you do?

Rank in order from 1 to 5 the following actions in response to this situation. Where 1 is the most appropriate action and 5 is the least appropriate action.

A. Contact the GMC. Patients are at risk and you need to do something about it immediately.

B. Do nothing. You have already informed the Consultant so there is little else you can do.

C. Seek advice from another Consultant who you feel comfortable speaking to.

D. Discuss the matter with the Clinical Director of the hospital.

E. Contact the media and expose the issue.

Question 50

You are on your way to your A&E night shift but are running slightly late as you have been stuck in traffic. You have called to say you are only ten minutes away. Whilst driving you notice a road traffic accident and the police are present but there is no ambulance. What do you do?

Rank in order from 1 to 5 the following actions in response to this situation. Where 1 is the most appropriate action and 5 is the least appropriate action.

A. Find a place to park your car immediately and attend the accident to offer your medical assistance.

B. Ignore what you have seen and keep on driving to the hospital to start your shift.

C. Stop temporarily and ask the police if they need your assistance.

D. Dial 999 and call for an ambulance.

E. Offer to drive the victims of the accident to A&E as you are on your way there anyway.

Question 51

You are a foundation doctor in hospital medicine and have recently started the post. You have noticed that during your Consultant ward rounds your Consultant does not seem to be following infection control procedures and is not washing their hands in between examining patients. What do you do?

Rank in order from 1 to 5 the following actions in response to this situation. Where 1 is the most appropriate action and 5 is the least appropriate action.

A. Nothing. It is not a serious issue and you do not wish to rock the boat.

B. Mention to the patients that they have the right to ask a doctor to wash their hands before examining them.

C. Inform the Clinical Director of the hospital

D. Discuss the matter with another Consultant

E. Discuss the matter politely with the Consultant in question.

Question 52

You have just arrived on hospital grounds for your eight hour shift that starts at midday. You have 15 minutes until your shift starts but can feel a migraine coming on. You get these frequently and usually take sumatriptan as they can be quite severe, but you have forgotten it. What do you do?

Rank in order from 1 to 4 the following actions in response to this situation. Where 1 is the most appropriate action and 4 is the least appropriate action.

A. Write yourself a quick prescription and go to the nearest pharmacy which is a few minutes away.

B. Telephone your GP to see if he would do a prescription for you that you could collect later when ready.

C. Start your shift and take some sumatriptan from the ward pharmacy cupboard hoping that no one notices.

D. Call in sick.

Question 53

You are in the middle of a busy 12 hour day shift when you realise you forgot to bring your insulin with you (you are a Type 1 Diabetic) which you will need for your afternoon meal. What do you do?

Rank in order from 1 to 5 the following actions in response to this situation. Where 1 is the most appropriate action and 5 is the least appropriate action.

A. Call your GP to see if he is able to do a prescription for you and fax it across to a neighbouring outside pharmacy for you to collect.

B. See if the insulin you take is available on the ward and ask one of the nurses to administer some to you.

C. Write a prescription for yourself and go to an outside pharmacy, leaving your bleep with one of your colleagues.

D. Call a relative at home to see if they can bring the insulin to the hospital for you.

E. Book yourself into A&E and get a prescription for the insulin that way.

Question 54

Whilst taking blood from a patient on the ward you sustain a needle-stick injury. You are quite concerned as the patient is an intravenous drug-user and you cannot remember when your last hepatitis B booster was. You are now being bleeped by your Registrar who is asking you to join both him and the Consultant for the afternoon ward round. What do you do?

Rank in order from 1 to 5 the following actions in response to this situation. Where 1 is the most appropriate action and 5 is the least appropriate action.

A. Go straight to the ward round and then come back to the ward later to consent and bleed the patient for a serum save.

B. Ask a medical student to consent and bleed the patient for a serum save whilst you are attending the ward round.

C. Explain to your Registrar what has happened and inform him that you are unable to attend the ward round straight away as you need to go to the Occupational Health department and arrange for the patient to be bled.

D. Quickly explain to the patient that you need to obtain his consent to bleed him immediately to screen for infections because you have sustained a needle stick injury, however you may not be able to answer all his questions now as you are needed on the ward round.

E. Ask the senior sister on the ward to deal with arranging the patient to be consented and bled whilst you attend the ward round.

Question 55

You have arranged to go out to dinner with your partner tonight as it is your anniversary. Just before leaving the ward your Consultant asks you if you would mind doing a presentation for the Grand Round tomorrow, as the person who is meant to be doing it has called in sick. What do you do?

Rank in order from 1 to 5 the following actions in response to this situation. Where 1 is the most appropriate action and 5 is the least appropriate action.

A. Agree to do the presentation but come in early the next day to complete it so that you can still attend dinner with your partner.

B. Explain to the Consultant that you have made plans with your partner and therefore are unable to prepare an adequate presentation in time for tomorrow.

C. Agree to do the presentation but ask one of your colleagues to help you with it explaining to them that you have dinner plans so you won't be able to do much.

D. Agree to do the presentation and cancel dinner with your partner.

E. Tell the Consultant a lie as to why you cannot do the presentation as you do not feel he will be sympathetic if you tell him the truth about your dinner plans.

Question 56

You are a FY2 doctor on a general practice rotation. A slightly overweight patient comes to you asking for an anti-obesity drug as she is having difficulty losing weight. Unfortunately her BMI does not fit the criteria for being eligible to have the drug and as she is just slightly overweight you do not feel comfortable giving her medication. What do you do?

Rank in order from 1 to 5 the following actions in response to this situation. Where 1 is the most appropriate action and 5 is the least appropriate action.

A. Advise her that her BMI is not high enough for her to be eligible for the drug, but if she should put on more weight in the future then she can come back for the medication.

B. Advise her that her BMI is not high enough to be eligible for the medication but she can buy it from the internet which is an option as she will be unable to get it on the NHS.

C. Give her the medication as she has honestly tried several diets and it will not do any harm for her to have the medication outside its licensed use.

D. Explain to her sensitively why you feel it is not in her best interests to have the medication but try to discuss other ways in which she could try to lose weight.

E. Explain to her why it is not in her best interest to have the medication but offer her a second opinion from another colleague if she wishes.

Question 57

One of your patients was due in court last week as he was on trial but did not attend. He asks you to backdate a sick note (MED3) for last week that he can show to the courts to certify he was unwell and not fit to attend. He claims that he had a bad cold and was in bed for the whole of that week. He did not see or call a doctor at that time. He does however have signs of an URTI today. What do you do?

Rank in order from 1 to 4 the following actions in response to this situation. Where 1 is the most appropriate action and 4 is the least appropriate action.

A. Explain to him that legally you cannot backdate a sick note but you will write a letter explaining that he was unwell at the time he was due to attend court.

B. Explain to him that in view of the fact that he did not contact a doctor during this illness you cannot verify he could not attend court and subsequently cannot sign any document saying he was unfit to attend court.

C. In view of the circumstance you backdate a sick certificate from last week to cover the patient when he did not attend court as he clearly has signs of a URTI today.

D. Explain to him that you cannot backdate a certificate nor can you certify that he was unwell to attend his court appointment as you did not see him during his illness. You can write a letter to the court stating that he is clearly unwell today and see whether this may support his testimony that he was unwell last week.

Question 58

Whilst on the ward round you overhear one of the Registrars talking to a patient in a sexual manner and from the conversation you suspect they are having a sexual relationship. What do you do next?

Rank in order from 1 to 5 the following actions in response to this situation. Where 1 is the most appropriate action and 5 is the least appropriate action.

A. Confront the Registrar there and then on the ward telling him that it is not appropriate for him to be engaging in a sexual relationship with any of his patients.
B. Call the GMC and inform them of the incident.
C. Seek advice from one of your more senior colleagues.
D. Tell the patient that the Registrar is wrong for having a sexual relationship with her and you will be taking this further.
E. Ask some of the other members of your team whether they are aware of the relationship and try to find out some more details.

Question 59

One of your patients has recently been diagnosed with epilepsy having had several fits in the past few months and has been on anti-convulsant medication for the past month. You have clearly informed him that he should not drive and that he needs to inform the DVLA. He has continued to drive despite you telling him not to and has told you that he intends to continue to drive regardless. What do you do?

Rank in order from 1 to 5 the following actions in response to this situation. Where 1 is the most appropriate action and 5 is the least appropriate action.

A. Tell him you will ring his wife and tell her that he is ignoring your advice if he continues to drive as it is unsafe for him and the public.
B. Tell him that you have no other choice but to inform the DVLA as he is ignoring your advice and still continuing to drive.
C. Try to persuade him not to drive and ask for his permission to discuss this matter with his wife.
D. Discuss the reasons why he is ignoring your advice about not driving and inform him that he is entitled to a second opinion from another doctor. Inform him that he should not drive however until he has that opinion.
E. Say nothing at the time but then contact the DVLA once the patient has left.

Question 60

One of your patients has recently been diagnosed with HIV whilst as an inpatient at your hospital. He asks you to withhold this information from his discharge summary to his GP as he does not want his GP to know about it. What do you do?

Rank in order from 1 to 5 the following actions in response to this situation. Where 1 is the most appropriate action and 5 is the least appropriate action.

A. Respect his wishes without any further question. The diagnosis of HIV does not need to be recorded in the discharge summary and thus you do not record it if the patient does not consent.

B. Explain to him the importance of recording his diagnosis in his notes and explain to him that his GP is unlikely to be able to provide the necessary care unless he knows his diagnosis. Also explain to him that this information will only be used by healthcare professionals and would not be released to anyone else without his consent. However, if he still declines accept his wishes.

C. Accept his request to withhold the information but then record the diagnosis on the discharge summary anyway, as you feel his GP needs to know.

D. Explain to him that you need to inform his GP as he poses a serious infection risk to the GP and staff at the practice, and therefore they need to know his status. Thus if he does not consent you will need to break his confidentiality in the best interests of the health and safety of his GP and practice staff.

E. Tell the patient that you have no choice but to record the information in his discharge summary, as you have an obligation to record accurate notes. Thus if he agrees or not you will be letting his GP know about his status.

Question 61

You are an FY2 doctor in a general practice rotation. A mother comes to see you with her six year old daughter who she is concerned about. She is going through a messy divorce and custody battle. She feels her daughter is not handling it well and would like her to see a psychologist. She asks you however to not put any documentation of the consultation in her daughter's notes as she is worried that her ex-husband will use it against her in court. She then becomes tearful. What do you do?

Rank in order from 1 to 5 the following actions in response to this situation. Where 1 is the most appropriate action and 5 is the least appropriate action.

A. Tell her that that you will not release the notes without her permission, even if a judge asks you to, so she does not need to worry.

B. Explain to her that you can understand why she is concerned but that it is important for other doctors in the practice to be aware that her daughter is having difficulties so they can provide her with the best care possible.

C. Agree not to enclose the information in her daughter's notes if she is adamant not to.

D. Comfort the mother and tell her that she is doing the best thing for her daughter by getting help.

E. Encourage her to tell her ex-husband about the referral to the psychologist to avoid it coming out in court.

Question 62

You are consulting with a young Asian patient who speaks no English. You have an interpreter present but you are slightly concerned that she is not translating exactly what you are saying. You are finding that when you ask a simple question she seems to take a lot of time to explain the question, and when the patient replies with a detailed response she gives you a very short answer. What do you do?

Rank in order from 1 to 5 the following actions in response to this situation. Where 1 is the most appropriate action and 5 is the least appropriate action.

A. End the consultation and rebook the patient with a different interpreter, as long as there is no serious medical issue that needs to be addressed immediately.

B. See if there is a different interpreter available, even if over the telephone, as you are not happy to continue with the interpreter.

C. Confront the interpreter in front of the patient with your complaint and ask her to translate exactly what is being said, and then continue with the consultation.

D. Continue with the consultation but have a private conversation with the interpreter afterwards voicing your complaints, and never book her again.

E. Do nothing. As you do not understand the language you cannot really prove your suspicions.

Question 63

You are a foundation doctor in your weekly 'bleep-free' teaching. Unfortunately you forgot to check your bleep in with the receptionist at the post-graduate centre and it is now going off. It is your ward bleeping you. What do you do?

Rank in order from 1 to 5 the following actions in response to this situation. Where 1 is the most appropriate action and 5 is the least appropriate action.

A. Ignore it. You are in a 'bleep-free' teaching where you should not be disturbed. Hopefully your ward will remember this and bleep someone else if you do not answer.

B. Ask one of your colleagues who is with you in the teaching session to answer your bleep for you and say you are not available.

C. Go straight to the ward to see who has bleeped you and what the matter is.

D. Answer the bleep explaining that you are in a 'bleep free' teaching at the moment and ask if they could bleep someone else on your team such as the SHO.

E. Answer the bleep and leave teaching immediately if you are required for any jobs on the ward.

Question 64

You are a junior doctor working on a gynaecological firm. It is a Friday evening and you have just seen an obviously mature and Gillick competent 15 year old pregnant patient with severe Hyperemesis Gravidarum. She needs to be admitted for IV fluids and further investigation. She is refusing to stay however as she does not want her mother to find out that she is pregnant. What do you do?

Rank in order from 1 to 5 the following actions in response to this situation. Where 1 is the most appropriate action and 5 is the least appropriate action.

A. Encourage her to stay explaining that it is in her best interest. Suggest that if she is worried about her mother finding out perhaps she could make up an excuse as to her whereabouts.

B. Explain to her that the details around her pregnancy are confidential and no one will release that information against her wishes. Thus if she stays the team will do their best to ensure that the details around her pregnancy are kept confidential.

C. Ignore her wishes as she is under age. Subsequently you are making the decision as to what is in her best interests and that is to remain as an inpatient for treatment.

D. Let her self-discharge without any discussion. She is entitled to leave if she wishes.

E. Encourage her to stay explaining to her that it is in her best interests. Suggest that perhaps she should tell her mother she is pregnant as she is likely to find out at some point in the future, and she may benefit from her mother's support at this time.

Question 65

You are a gynaecological FY2 doctor and a 12 year old has been admitted with abdominal pain. She is subsequently diagnosed with PID. On further questioning you determine she has been having a sexual relationship with a 14 year old boy from her school. What do you do?

Rank in order from 1 to 5 the following actions in response to this situation. Where 1 is the most appropriate action and 5 is the least appropriate action.

A. Assess whether this was consensual sex and that she is competent to make a decision to enter into a sexual relationship. If satisfied with this then you simply advise her on safe sex and contraception.

B. Call the boy's parents and inform them about what has happened.

C. Inform her parents about the relationship and let them handle the situation. It is not your duty to get involved or tell her parents what to do.

D. Call the police.

E. Discuss the case with the child protection lead of the hospital.

Chapter 5 Situational Judgement Tests: Practice Answers

Question 1
Answer: 1.D 2.E 3.B 4.C 5.A

This is a scenario which assesses several qualities. It mainly assesses your empathy and communication skills but also how you problem solve. The main dilemma is that a criminal offence has occurred and you need to use your common sense in how to deal with the matter promptly but sensitively. When dealing with these scenarios it is useful to start by determining the facts. You can they make a decision on whether to inform any others depending on the severity of the crime. You should always aim to only involve the appropriate people and deal with the matter locally first.

Option D: Reading the scenarios there is one option that seems the most appropriate to start with. Option D actually establishes the details of what has happened whilst comforting the patient at the same time. Although such a large scale theft is a criminal offence and you are likely to need to involve the police, you will need to establish the details and be sure the laptop and wallet are truly missing. Thus Option D is the most appropriate action.

Option A: The least appropriate action that stands out is Option A. Although asking other patients if they have seen anything may seem at first like a sensible idea, this may be interpreted as you accusing them of the theft, especially if you start searching their cabinets. This is likely to just cause panic and chaos and cause great offence by making the patients feel like a criminal. Thus Option A is the least appropriate action.

You are then left with three options. One of these options involves involving someone more senior and involving the police. The remaining two options involve doing something to try and ensure that this incident does not happen again.

Option E: As stated in Chapter 2, you should try to prioritise options that involve taking immediate action over those that involve dealing with the matter later. Speaking to the senior nurse in charge and calling the police is likely to be more helpful and beneficial than taking steps to prevent it again. It also seems a sensible idea now that you have the details around the theft. Thus Option E is the 2nd most appropriate action.

Options B and C: You are then left with either filling in a critical incident form or putting up posters around the ward to ensure that everyone is more vigilant. Both of these actions would bring the alleged theft to the attention of others and would try to prevent it from happening. Although by putting up posters around the ward, you are bringing the theft to everyone's attention, it is not the most subtle way to do it and may distress other patients or relatives and instil fear. By filling in an incident form you are able to hand over the investigation of the incident to more senior colleagues who may then be able to put certain mechanisms in place to lessen the risk of any future thefts. Thus Option B is more appropriate than Option C and is the 3rd most appropriate action. This leaves Option C as the 4th most appropriate action.

Partial mark answer

There really aren't many partial mark variants to this question. Only three options (A, D and E) involve addressing the theft immediately and out of these Option A is obviously inappropriate and should be ranked last. Logically it does not make sense to inform the senior sister without actually obtaining any concrete details first and thus it would not be appropriate to place Option E before Option D, although you wouldn't lose too many marks if you had done so. It should also be clear as to why Option B ranked before Option C, however had you ranked these two the other way round you would have still gained partial marks as long as the other options were ranked correctly.

Question 2
Answer: 1.C 2.E 3.A 4.B 5.D

This scenario is similar to the previous question and assesses both your professional integrity and how you work with colleagues. You have a duty to not ignore what you have seen especially as it may involve conduct issues in another colleague. However, you do not have to deal with this situation alone. If it is handled incorrectly it may destroy your working relationship with your colleague as well as the trust of the patient in the profession.

Option D: The least appropriate action here is Option D. Although theft is a criminal offence it is not always necessary to call the police as previously stated. You need to assess the severity of the crime and the facts well before involving others, especially the police. This is a minor theft, and most importantly you have no evidence that your colleague stole the watch so to call the police would be inappropriate, especially for the first action.

Option C: Conversely, the most appropriate action is Option C. This is because it involves you dealing with the matter tactfully and trying to gather the facts before assuming that your colleague stole the watch and involving others. It also gives your colleague the chance to explain themselves before you assume the worst.

Options A and B: These two options are not ideal. Both of these options involve assuming the worst and confronting your colleague with little evidence. To confront your colleague publicly in front of everyone without establishing the facts is inappropriate and you would probably be way out of your depth in doing so. You are immediately making an accusation without establishing the facts. However, to make the assumption that your colleague stole the watch and then relay that to the patient is even more inappropriate. Not only do you not have any evidence but if you are wrong you may have distressed the patient and in the process destroyed their trust in the medical profession. Thus Option B is the 2nd least appropriate action and Option C is the 3rd least appropriate action.

Option E: Involving a senior may be a little drastic in view of the fact that you have very little evidence, however this option seems more appropriate than the other options discussed. By informing a senior of what you have seen you are allowing them to investigate the matter further and this has to be better than accusing your colleague in front of everyone, calling the police or telling the patient you think that a colleague stole his watch. Thus Option E is the 2nd most appropriate action.

Partial Marks

Had you ranked Option E before Option C (i.e. ECABD), choosing immediately to gain senior help instead of discussing it with your colleague you would have scored partial marks. It is a delicate situation and it may be one you would not feel comfortable with at all. However, there may be a really simple explanation, and to go straight to the Consultant without even letting your colleague explain themselves may lead to embarrassment and distress for your colleague. Option C was therefore ranked as the most appropriate option in the model answer.

Question 3
Answer: 1.D 2.B 3.A 4.E 5.C

This is another question assessing how you work with colleagues but also looks at your professional integrity. The ethical dilemma here is that of protecting your patients together with respecting your colleagues. Although it is your senior who seems to be struggling, and you may feel uncomfortable dealing with it, you must not ignore the situation. This is because as stated, we must never ignore any near misses or potential patient safety issues. Although it may have only been a simple error that has occurred it has been one of many. If you continue to ignore the issue there may be a day when a much larger error is made and a patient put at serious risk. Thus you have a duty to protect the safety of your patients and to inform someone if you feel patient safety may be compromised. On the other hand, you also have a duty to be sensitive and respectful to your colleagues. Your Consultant may simply be having personal problems and going through a bad patch away from work, and you need to be empathetic towards that and not go overboard. In view of this the most and least appropriate actions are clear.

Option C: The least appropriate action must be Option C. Approaching the GMC when only a simple error has been made is not only an exaggerated response but could also be viewed as undermining your colleague. You have not showed any sensitivity towards your colleague by doing so and are not even allowing him the opportunity to address the matter himself. In addition the GMC should only be involved as a last resort, when addressing the matter locally has failed. Option C is therefore entirely inappropriate.

Option D: The most appropriate action is Option D. Here you are acknowledging that there may be a problem, but you are aware that as a junior doctor you may not be the best person to deal with it alone. Therefore it seems reasonable to address your concerns with a senior colleague. This approach not only addresses the issue but also allows you to obtain a second opinion of whether the matter needs to be taken any further.

Option E: This seems to be the least appropriate action out of the remaining option. The nurse on the ward is not in a position with regards to her role to address this issue any more than you are. Thus informing her of all the errors your Consultant has made and of your concerns is unlikely to be beneficial at all.

By involving her in this issue, you could be seen as creating rumour and gossip, and again it is unlikely to resolve the issue at hand. You may also be seen as putting the responsibility onto another junior colleague which shows lack of courtesy or respect for your colleague. Thus Option E is the least beneficial out of the remaining options and is the 2nd least appropriate action.

Options A and B: You are now left with two options: one of which involves dealing with the matter immediately by talking to your Consultant and the other involves filling an incident form which would delay handling the matter. Filling in an incident form is also unlikely to really address the issue and get to the bottom of what may be causing your Consultant's dip in performance. Also as it may take some time for the incident to be addressed and patients are potentially at risk it is not as appropriate as taking immediate action. Although talking to the Consultant yourself may not be the most appropriate action, and is probably something most of us would feel uncomfortable with, it is at least addressing the issue. Thus Option B ranks above Option A and is the 2nd most appropriate action. This leaves Option A ranked 3rd.

Partial marks

Some of you may have felt it better to go to your Consultant immediately before discussing the matter with someone else (i.e. ranked BDAEC). This could be appropriate because you are demonstrating that you realise you need to take immediate action. However, as we are answering these questions from the perspective of a foundation doctor it is probably more appropriate to discuss it with another senior who we feel comfortable with. This is likely to be less threatening than going to your Consultant directly and probably more beneficial.

Also, many of you may not have felt comfortable with ranking talking to your Consultant as the 2nd most appropriate answer and perhaps felt more comfortable filling in an incident form before doing this (i.e. DABEC). Although this is understandable, filling in an incident form is not dealing with the situation immediately and as patients could be at risk the situation must be addressed. Thus although you would have scored marks for ranking the other options correctly you would not gain many marks for this approach.

Question 4
Answer: B, E and G

This is a common scenario in A&E and tests your professional integrity. Alcoholic patients that are inebriated can often be very difficult to manage especially when they clearly need medical attention but decline. It can be a situation where you feel uncomfortable, unsafe and may have certain feelings and attitudes towards these patients that can hinder their care. The GMC clearly states in Good Medical Practice that:

'*You must not refuse or delay treatment because you believe that a patient's actions have contributed to their condition. You must treat your patients with respect whatever their life choices and beliefs. You must not unfairly discriminate against them by allowing your personal views to affect adversely your professional relationship with them or the treatment you provide or arrange*'.

Therefore, although this patient is inebriated and verbally aggressive, and this is of his own accord, it is not a reason to refuse to treat the patient. He is inebriated and is unlikely to understand the severity of his injuries, thus although he is saying he does not want to see a doctor, you should at least attempt to explain his injuries to him.

Option C and D: In view of this, Options C and D are not appropriate actions to take. You cannot simply refuse to see him because of your personal feelings towards alcoholic patients nor can you refuse to see him because he says he does not want a doctor when he clearly has injuries and is not in full faculties to make that decision. You should at least attempt to attend to the patient. You do however have to consider your own safety in all of this. Thus you need to make the situation as safe as possible when reviewing this patient. In view of this there are certain options that seem sensible.

Option A: Here you ask another colleague who is more senior to deal with the situation protecting your own personal safety. However this is not ideal as you are passing the responsibility onto another colleague. This does not show good team work. Also, just because a colleague is more senior in their experience, it does not make them any more secure in this situation than you. Thus Option A is not an ideal action.

Option G: This is a better alternative. Here you inform your senior that you are slightly worried for your safety when seeing this patient, and ask for help and support. There is a difference between asking someone else to see the patient where you would be passing on the responsibility and asking someone else to be present for safety reasons whilst you fulfil your duties. Hence Option G is a suitable action to take.

Option B: This again seems sensible in that we are attending to the patient but have someone present in case any trouble occurs. Hospital security is used to these kinds of situations and would be the ideal staff to have present in case of any trouble arising. Thus Option B is a sensible action.

Option E: Similarly trying to calm down the patient verbally is a suitable option. Regardless of whether someone is inebriated or not, talking to someone calmly and professionally can often diffuse situations. Alcoholic or not, he still deserves the same courtesy as anyone else and a simple explanation that you just want to examine his head injury may calm him down. However, if this does not work and he continues to be abusive to you and refuses to let you examine him, you are well within your rights to not attend to the patient. However, you must document this clearly.

Option F: Although this may allow you to treat the patient quickly it is not ethical to sedate a patient against his wishes neither is it safe in this circumstance. The patient is already inebriated and suffering from a head injury, thus to sedate the patient is unsafe as you would not be able to check for any deterioration in his condition. Option F is therefore entirely inappropriate.

Question 5
Answer: 1.D 2.C 3.E 4.B 5.A
This question once again assesses your professional integrity which can be described as your willingness to be accountable for your own actions. Ultimately you are responsible to check the expiry date before giving the vaccination and thus you are responsible for the error. The GMC states that if you do make an error with a patient you must:

'act immediately to put matters right, if that is possible. You should offer an apology and explain fully and promptly to the patient what has happened and the likely short-term and long-term effects'.

Thus, you need to address the issue, and explain to the mother what has happened. Although, nothing serious may happen from the expired injection, the child may not be protected as the vaccine was out of date.

Option A: Option A is inappropriate as it involves being dishonest and not admitting the error as well as the false belief that it does not matter if the vaccine is out of date. Thus you are lying to the mother about the error as well as putting the child at risk by covering up the mistake. Option A is therefore the least appropriate action to take.

Option B: Although this involves being honest about the mistake, to falsely reassure the mother is unsafe. In addition, the option states that you 'have a feeling' that it should still be okay, and it would be wrong to falsely reassure the mother on nothing but a hunch. If you are not sure of the consequences of giving an expired vaccine, then you should at least ask advice from a senior, before reassuring the mother. Also as previously stated, the child may be at risk as the vaccine may have not been effective. Option B is the 2nd least appropriate action. It is slightly better than Option A in that at least you admit to the error, although in both options the potential harm to the child is not addressed.

We are now left with various ways to deal with the situation correctly and these should be ranked in priority of the manner and the speed with which they address the situation.

Option D: This has to be the most appropriate action to take. Not only does it involve admitting the mistake and acting with honesty and integrity, but also addresses the situation immediately. As you may not be sure on what to do in this situation, by obtaining senior help immediately you are ensuring that the child is safe and any questions or concerns the mother may have are addressed immediately. Option D is therefore the most appropriate action.

Options C and E: These options are both sensible actions to take and are far more appropriate than doing nothing or being dishonest to the mother. By ensuring that the vaccines in the fridge are in date, you are ensuring to some degree that this does not happen again in the immediate future. By also discussing it as a significant event at the next practice meeting you are also looking at ways to avoid the event from happening in the future. However, checking the vaccines in the fridge is more appropriate in that it is taking more immediate action to prevent the incident from occurring again. Thus Option C ranks before Option E and these options are the 2nd and 3rd most appropriate actions respectively.

Question 6
Answer: B and E
This question is similar to the previous scenario and so once again addresses your professional integrity. It also assesses your ability to problem solve as you are put in a difficult situation. However, you must remember the ethics behind patient safety in this question and must act with honesty and integrity. Although you may feel awkward that the patient has waited to see you and you are not trained to do the procedure, you should not attempt to do a procedure that you are not competent in. Not only could this result in local complications for the patient e.g. infection, it may also result in loss of contraceptive efficacy that could be catastrophic for the patient.

Options A and C: It is unsafe and unethical to give the injection regardless of whether you inform the patient of your lack of experience or not. Obviously it is even more unethical to pretend to be competent to a patient, but either way you should not give the injection. Thus Options A and C are inappropriate.

Option E: This seems like a reasonable action to take. Although your colleagues may be busy and tell you to rebook the patient you have nothing to lose by asking if someone could come and given her the injection. It is unlikely to take much time to do so and you would be able to witness how to give the injection for your learning purposes. Obviously, if someone is able to give her the injection now you would negate the need for the patient to rebook, and thus Option E is appropriate.

You are now left with two choices: either send the patient straight to A&E to have the injection or ask the patient to rebook.

Options B and D: Sending the patient to A&E seems slightly drastic and would be an inappropriate referral. If anything it would seem more sensible to advise the patient to go to a family planning clinic which would be a more suitable place to receive the Depo injection. The patient has already waited to see you and may have a long wait in A&E. As it is not a life or death situation it seems more appropriate to ask her to rebook to see one of the other doctors or the nurse. Thus Option B is appropriate whereas Option D is not.

Partial Marks
There is not a partial mark answer to this question that would be considered a reasonable alternative to the model answer. However, some of you may have felt that as her contraceptive injection is due that it is safer to send her to A&E than to rebook her to see someone else in case she cannot get an appointment. Although it may be the case that the appointments are full it is reading a little too much into the question. We are not given any details on how overdue the injection is or the appointment state of the practice. It seems more sensible to ask her to come back to the surgery at a convenient time than to send her to A&E unnecessarily. Thus Option D is not an appropriate action.

Question 7
Answer: B and D
This question deals with assessing your communication skills and your professional integrity. Once again there is specific GMC guidance on prescribing which states that:

'you should only prescribe drugs to meet identified needs of patients and never for your own convenience or simply because patients demand them'.

In this circumstance the patient does not meet the necessary requirements for primary prevention with a statin and thus if you did prescribe it, it would literally be because the patient was demanding it and not because it was in their best interest. Also one has to remember that as a general practitioner you are a gate keeper to NHS resources and you have a duty to ration the services appropriately. One could argue that by prescribing an unnecessary medication to a patient who does not need it you are subsequently now making less resources available to others who may truly require medication for their health and well-being.

However, on the other hand the patient does have a right to decide what they feel is best for them. Thus you do need to listen to the patient and respect their views. If you do not feel a particular treatment is right for them you should communicate with them and explain to the patient why you feel the way you do, but you must attempt to address their concerns. The GMC guidance on this is:

'If the patient asks for a treatment that the doctor considers would not be of overall benefit to them, the doctor should discuss the issues with the patient and explore the reasons for their request. If, after discussion, the doctor still considers that the treatment would not be of overall benefit to the patient, they do not have to provide the treatment. But they should explain their reasons to the patient, and explain any other options that are available, including the option to seek a second opinion'.

In view of this there are a few options that are not the most appropriate actions to take.

Option E: To simply refuse to prescribe the statin without explaining to the patient the reasons why you are refusing is not appropriate. It does not show good communication skills and is likely to harm the doctor-patient relationship. We should always involve patients in treatment decisions and listen to their concerns, thus we must never refuse a patient's request without an explanation. Thus Option E is inappropriate.

Option C: Although we do have a responsibility to take patient's own views into consideration when making management decisions, according to the GMC, we should not compromise our own clinical judgement just to suit a patient's demands. Thus to simply back down because the patient is demanding a particular prescription, even though you do not feel the treatment is in their best interest is not acceptable. Thus Option C is not appropriate.

Option A: Along similar lines Option A is not appropriate either. Not only are we giving a patient something that we feel not to be in their best interest, we are now passing the responsibility onto another colleague. You should address the issue immediately with the patient, instead of prescribing it and asking them to come back to see another colleague, who you hope will decline a further prescription. Your other colleague is also likely to have even more difficulty in persuading the patient that they do not need a statin when you have already prescribed it and this shows poor teamwork. Thus Option A is not appropriate.

We have already mentioned that the correct way of dealing with this situation is to explain to the patient why you do not feel a statin is appropriate and the remaining two options involve doing this in various ways.

Option B: This seems like a reasonable approach to take. Here we try to take the patient's views and concerns into consideration and explain to them why we feel the statin is not in their best interest. A simple explanation of how statins work and why they are not needed in his case may allow the patient to understand that a statin is really not in his best interest. This is the recommended approach and therefore seems like an appropriate action to take.

Option D: In this option we explain to the patient our reasons behind why we are reluctant to prescribe a statin but offer the patient a second opinion if he so wishes. By doing this we are empowering the patient and giving him alternative options, however we are not backing down when we really feel that to prescribe a statin would not be in his best interest. Thus Option D is also appropriate.

Question 8
Answer: 1.B 2.A 3.D 4.E 5.C

As this is a question on working with others and involves the conduct of another colleague we can ask the necessary questions that we discussed in Chapter 2: is there an issue at hand; is there a patient safety or legal issue and is there sufficient evidence to support the allegation? In this situation there is clearly an issue at hand, and patient safety could have been compromised by the lack of sufficient cover. It also shows poor teamwork and needs to be addressed. The GMC states that:

'Patient care may be compromised if there is not sufficient medical cover. There-
fore, you must take up any post, including a locum post, you have formally
accepted, and you must work your contractual notice period, unless the
employer has reasonable time to make other arrangements'.

Although, calling in sick is acceptable if you are truly unwell, to do so at the last minute based on dishonesty is not acceptable. On the other hand you are unsure of your colleague's reasons for doing so, and as stated in Chapter 2, should also show some empathy towards your fellow colleague.

Option C: As we have already stated that there is an issue at hand and it could have potentially been a patient safety issue, to do nothing is not an option. Thus Option C is the least appropriate action.

We now have four options left: three of which involve dealing with the situation immediately and the other involves postponing addressing the issue until our next appraisal.

Option E: This is inappropriate as it involves delaying dealing with the issue at hand. In Chapter 2 we discussed that in general we should aim to rank options that involve dealing with the situation immediately above those that involve delaying the matter. Your next appraisal may be several months away and the problem may continue if you do not address it immediately. In addition, your appraisal is to discuss your progress and it is not the correct forum in which to discuss problems with other colleagues. Thus Option E is the 2nd least appropriate action to take. It is obviously slightly better than doing nothing and hence Option C is still the least appropriate action.

We are now left with the decision to inform management or someone senior or discuss the matter with our colleague.

Option B: This is the courteous approach to take. Although there could be a potential safety issue if this doctor keeps calling in sick at the last minute, no patient has actually been harmed and therefore it may be appropriate to try and discuss the matter with the doctor themselves. At least then we would be able to find out the reasons behind their actions (e.g. it mentions they did a locum at another hospital so they could possibly be having financial problems) and allow them a chance to defend themselves or rectify the situation. Thus Option B is the most appropriate action.

Options A and D: We are now left with two options, all of which involve discussing the matter with someone senior. As we have stated before it is best initially to deal with the matter locally and thus it would make more sense to inform the consultant first instead of medical personnel. Thus Option A is the 2nd most appropriate action to take leaving Option D to rank 3rd.

Partial mark answer

Had you felt more comfortable talking to medical personnel for various reasons (i.e. ranked BDAEC) you would have scored partial marks as Options D and A, are very similar. The majority of the marks are given for realising that to do nothing is not an option and for attempting to address the matter with your colleague yourself before involving seniors (i.e. ranking Option B and Option C in the correct place). However, as it makes more logical sense, to involve those closer to the team, the model answer ranks Option A before Option D.

Question 9
Answer: C, E and F

This question assesses your professional integrity and your personal values, as well as your communication skills. We have discussed the approach to accepting gifts in great detail in Chapter 2. As you may remember the key to answering the question is to ask yourself whether you feel comfortable or not with the gift and the situation. Gifts are a grey area but in general if the gift seems appropriate for the level of service and you do not feel that the patient feels pressured or coerced into giving you gifts, there is not an issue. You do need to be careful when accepting gifts and make sure you can defend yourself if your intentions are questioned.

Initially, when you were given the first gift you probably did not think much of it. As you had taken care of her when she was quite unwell, a box of chocolates as a thank you gift does not seem untoward. However, the fact that this person constantly brings you a gift during your routine appointments should raise some degree of suspicion, even if it turns out to be for a completely innocent reason.

Option A: Based on what we have discussed Option A is not the best action from the seven available. Here we have a patient who received good clinical care and was appreciative of that but now, perhaps, may feel obliged to keep on giving gifts in order to receive that. Thus to simply accept the gift without even considering this is not appropriate. The question clearly states that she brings you gifts every time she sees you for a routine appointment and although this may be innocent you need to at least consider the possibility that she feels somewhat obliged to do so.

Option B: On the other hand to refuse the gift informing the patient that people may get suspicious is rude and may affect your relationship with the patient. In this scenario you are making the patient feel guilty for the gift when she may have genuine intentions. Thus if you decide to refuse the gift you need to be more tactile in your approach. Thus Option B is not appropriate.

Options D and G: In these options you simply accept the chocolates from the patient without question, but then give them to others. This is not ideal as you are not addressing the issue and are not making it clear to the patient that although you are grateful, she does not need to keep giving you gifts to receive good care. Although you may ease your conscience slightly by not keeping the gift, you may still be perpetuating the patient's perception that she needs to give gifts in order to be treated by you.

By simply eliminating these answers first we are left with the most appropriate answers.

Option C: Here you try and enquire the reasons behind why she is giving you the gifts. Many elderly patients remember the old days when they had to pay to see a doctor and are just used to showing their gratitude that way. Thus with this option you are trying to ascertain whether she feels pressured into giving you a gift. By informing the patient that you are sharing the gift out with the team you are reminding her that her care is a team effort and are not taking all the glory for yourself. Thus Option C is appropriate.

Option F: Again with this option you are clearly explaining that she is not under any obligation to keep giving you gifts but acknowledge her feelings and the impact declining the gift may have on your relationship. If you do need to accept the gift by writing her a businesslike letter of thanks you are reminding her that this is a professional relationship and can avoid the relationship straying out of the correct boundaries.

Option E: This is similar to Option F but at the end you simply accept the gift if she insists. Although this is not ideal it is a more appropriate action than to accept the gift without any explanation that it is unnecessary (as stipulated in Options A, D and G) or refusing the gift quite abruptly and rudely as in Option B.

Thus the three most appropriate actions are Options C, E and F.

Question 10
Answer: A, C and D

Accepting gifts is a grey area and is designed to assess your professional and personal integrity. In general, you may accept gifts as long as you are not attempting or could be seen to be manipulating or abusing your relationship with the patient. This question is distinctively different from the previous question which also dealt with accepting a gift from a patient. Applying the rules we have learnt, a one-off gift of a few vegetables from an allotment, as is the case here, should not cause any concern.

Thus it would be appropriate to accept the gift if you felt comfortable in doing so. However, you should avoid giving any impression that gifts are necessary to continue their doctor-patient relationship with you as this would constitute abuse of that relationship. Also, you would be well within your rights to decline a gift if you did not feel comfortable with the situation. However, you should be sensitive in your approach and try not to offend the patient.

Option A: Accepting the gift without any question is appropriate here. It is a one-off gift and is appropriate in view of what the patient is claiming the gift is for. However, if the gift was very large or extravagant it may raise eyebrows and you should be more careful in accepting this sort of gift. Thus Option A is appropriate.

Options B and E: These options are not acceptable. Not because they involve declining the gift but in view of the manner in which they do so. To tell the patient that you cannot accept the gift as it may be seen as suspicious may come across as rude and the patient may feel guilty when they have really done nothing wrong. To decline the gift by telling the patient you 'don't like vegetables' is abrupt and likely to cause offence.

Option C: This is the only option that involves making sure the patient is aware that although you are grateful there really was no need to give you a gift. This is particularly important if you choose to accept the gift as it ensures that there are clear boundaries in place and that the patient feels in no way pressured to keep giving you gifts. Thus Option C is appropriate.

Option F: On the other hand to ask the patient to bring you some more vegetables next week may do just the opposite. This may reinforce to the patient that they need to keep you happy by giving you gifts in order to maintain the relationship and ensure good quality care should they become ill again. If this was the case it would be an abuse of the doctor-patient relationship and thus Option F is inappropriate.

Option D: Informing the patient that his care was a team effort and that you are going to share the gift with the team, is an excellent alternative to accepting the gift yourself. Again this is setting clear boundaries and ensuring that the situation could not possibly be misconstrued that you are influencing your patients to give you gifts and directly benefit yourself.

Option G: Although you may need to seek senior or specialist advice when accepting certain gifts, e.g. monetary gifts, a small gift of some vegetables in view of the circumstances hardly warrants discussing it with your Consultant. In view of the fact that there are more suitable options, Option G is not one of the three most appropriate actions.

Thus this leaves us with Option A, C and D as the three most appropriate actions.

Question 11
Answer: B, D and E
This question looks at how you work with colleagues and your ability to problem solve. It also addresses the ethics behind cover as well as the issue of trying to achieve a work/life balance. Thus, we need to balance our duty to ensure that we hand over correctly with our right to be able to have outside commitments. However, we must ensure that when we leave work our patients are safe and that all the necessary information needed to ensure this has been passed on to the relevant professionals. In addition, as our night colleague is doing us a favour by coming in early we must show some appreciation for that, even though they are late, and treat our colleague with respect.

Option A: To call up our colleague to have a go at them is not professional. We have no right to do so especially as they are doing us a favour by coming in early, which they did not have to agree to do. Thus we should try to remain calm and polite when enquiring the whereabouts of our colleague. Thus Option A is not appropriate.

Option G: Similarly, to ask your Registrar to call your colleague is not appropriate as it is treating the colleague as if they have done something wrong. Admittedly, they are late with regards to the agreed time you have for handover, but they are not late for their shift. Therefore to involve a senior at this stage is unnecessary and unfair to your colleague. Thus Option G is also not appropriate.

In Chapter 2, we discussed the GMC's guidance on cover. To reiterate we have a duty to ensure that we have effective handover arrangements involving clear communication with our colleagues, when going off duty. We can therefore eliminate obvious inappropriate actions that go against this guidance.

Option C: Although we are expected to have outside work commitments we must ensure our patient's safety. Thus to rush handover to get to our party is not appropriate as it is likely to cause miscommunication and therefore may put patients at risk.

Option F: Similarly handing over to a nurse is not appropriate and does not show good teamwork. The nurse is likely to feel out of her depth and you are now making her responsible for handing over the relevant information to the night doctor. Also it would be completely inappropriate to leave without there being another doctor to cover should there be any emergency, and you would be leaving the day Registrar alone which would be unsafe.

We are now left with three options which should be the most appropriate actions to take. However, you should always review these actions carefully and ensure they do not contradict each other.

Option D: In view of the fact that your colleague is not here yet and technically you should not leave until cover arrives, it is sensible to inform your friends that you may be slightly late.

Option E: This seems like a sensible compromise. Although ideally you should hand over to your colleague, the night Registrar will be looking after the same patients and therefore could pass on the details about the patients to your colleague. However, you recognise that you cannot just leave before your colleague arrives and leave the night Registrar alone. By calling to see where your colleague is you can therefore think of alternative arrangements if they are going to be late. By handing over to the night Registrar, but waiting until your colleague arrives before you leave, you are allowing yourself to get away as soon as your colleague arrives. However, you are not leaving the night Registrar alone which would be unsafe.

Option B: Although this option is not ideal as you may be late for your party, it is the responsible and sensible thing to do, and is more appropriate in view of the other options. You do have a responsibility to stay until your shift ends and you cannot simply leave without there being cover. As your colleague technically is not meant to start their shift for another 20 minutes, you cannot assume they are not coming, or ask others to find out their whereabouts. Thus you may just need to wait patiently until they arrive as the other options are unacceptable.

Thus Options B, D and E are the most appropriate actions to take.

Question 12
Answer: 1.C 2.A 3.E 4.B 5.D

This question is one where you have to think quickly on your feet. It also assesses your communication skills, empathy and your ability to problem solve. It represents a difficult situation where although you have a duty to listen to the relatives' complaints you need to be fair to your colleagues who are not there to answer for themselves. Thus you need to be careful in what you say and also in how you handle the situation. Saying the wrong thing or even not saying anything at all, could leave the relatives even more upset and could result in a complaint against your colleagues.

Although you have no knowledge regarding this patient and may not have enough information in the notes to understand why certain decisions were made, you do have angry relatives confronting you. You have a duty to try and diffuse the situation but you need to be honest when answering their questions and do so to the best of your ability. There may be questions that you are unable to answer and you should be honest in saying so. You also obviously need to be very careful in what you say as if you say the wrong thing it could make the situation worse.

Option C: In view of this Option C seems like a sensible action. Here you are dealing with the situation at hand, but are being honest in informing the relatives that you may not be able to fully answer their questions, as you can only go on what has been written in the notes. It may be the case that the reason for the patient still being on the ward is clearly documented, but it may also be the case that it is not, so you at least need to warn the relatives of this possibility. However, at least you are taking their concerns seriously and you are making some attempt to answer their questions. This is preferable to simply telling the patient's relatives that you are not looking after their relative and leaving them upset and angry without any answers. This is not best practice and does not show any empathy at all. It may also make the situation worse for your colleagues. Thus Option C is the most appropriate action.

Option D: In this option we do not address the relatives concerns at all and inform them to contact the PALS department in order to make a complaint. This does not show any professional courtesy for our colleagues nor does it show any empathy and sensitivity for the upset relatives. It may be that there is indeed a reason for them to make a formal complaint or it may simply be a misunderstanding. By not even attempting to address the matter in any other way you are now going to be partially responsible for a formal complaint against your colleagues. Although, it may be the case that the relatives ask you for details on how to make a complaint during your discussion anyway, this is not the case now. Thus it is entirely inappropriate to ignore the relatives and to basically tell them that if they are unhappy they should complain. Thus Option D is the least appropriate option.

Option B: This option also appears to be inappropriate. Although the nurse may know the patient better than you, the relatives have asked to speak to a doctor. They are angry and it would be entirely inappropriate to pass this responsibility onto the nurse. It would not show any professional courtesy for your colleague and is likely to just infuriate the relatives. It is slightly better however than just ignoring the relatives request to discuss the patient and telling them to make a formal complaint. Thus Option B is the 2nd least appropriate answer and ranks 4th.

You are now left with two options that are quite similar. On one hand you can explain to the relatives that as you do not normally look after the patient it may be best if they discuss their concerns with a member of the team tomorrow. On the other hand you can ring the Consultant looking after the patient to ask him how to answer these relatives questions here and now.

Options A and E: Although Option E where you call the Consultant may be dealing with the situation immediately, it does not come across as the most suitable option out of the two. The Consultant is not on call so technically speaking you are now calling him out of work hours for something that could be dealt with on another day. As this is not an issue technically over the clinical care of the patient there is no reason why this issue needs to be addressed completely today. Also, the Consultant does not have the patient's notes in front of him and to ask him to answer questions on the phone with you as the go-between is not the best way of handling the situation. It would be far more appropriate and professional for the family to have a meeting with the Consultant face to face. This would also give the team a chance to prepare for the meeting and read through the notes beforehand and would be fairer to your colleagues. It is also more likely to be beneficial for the relatives as the team would be better prepared to answer their questions. Thus Option E ranks after Option A as it is less appropriate. This makes Option A the 2nd most appropriate action and Option E the 3rd most appropriate.

Partial marks

You would have scored partial marks for asking the relatives to discuss their concerns with the team before trying to answer some of the questions yourself (i.e. ACEBD). Some of you may have felt worried that you may say the wrong thing and make the situation worse. Thus you may have felt it better to perhaps say nothing and let the team deal with it the next day. Although, you would be right in wanting to be careful about what you say, you cannot ignore the fact that you have angry and upset relatives. Therefore although you may feel uncomfortable or worried that you will say something wrong, you need to show a degree of responsibility. It may be that you are able to answer all the relatives' questions based on what is written in the notes and the complaint never materialises. Or it may be that you at least calm them down slightly which will be better than leaving them angry. In view of the fact that Option C clearly states that you inform the relatives that you may not be able to answer all their questions, you have at least covered yourself should you feel unable or uncomfortable answering certain questions. Thus you cannot truly condone not dealing with the situation at all which would not show any empathy for the upset relatives. Thus Option A is not as appropriate as Option C and did not feature first in the model answer.

For similar reasons some of you may have felt it better to contact the Consultant responsible first before trying to answer the relatives' questions yourself as he would be in a better position to answer the questions (i.e. ECABD). You may have also felt that if you could not answer the relatives' questions yourself that it was preferable to contact the Consultant than to delay dealing with the matter till tomorrow (i.e. CEABD). Those of you who did so may have remembered a similar question in the worked example chapter and felt it safer to address this issue now. The safest thing would be to speak to the Consultant first who would be able to answer the questions, or speak to him after if you could not answer the questions yourself.

Although you may have scored some marks for this approach you are unlikely to get a high number of marks. Unlike the example in Chapter 3, where the relatives were complaining about the clinical care of the patient, this issue is entirely different. There is unlikely to be an immediate patient safety issue involved in the patient not being discharged to the residential home. Contacting the Consultant out of hours first or if you are unable to answer the questions would not demonstrate any responsibility. This may have been different had the patient been very unwell or there was some evidence of gross negligence that needed to be immediately addressed. However as this is not the case it makes far more sense to try and answer as much as you could yourself, and then leave it to the team tomorrow if there were questions that remained unanswered.

Question 13
Answer: A and D

This question assesses your empathy and communication skills as well as your integrity. You may feel quite uncomfortable in this position where the patient is asking you such a direct and serious question, and you are unsure of the answer at this time. It is difficult to achieve a balance between not falsely reassuring the patient that cancer is unlikely but at the same time not convincing them that cancer is the only possibility. However, you do have a duty to be honest and give the patient the correct information. You should not tell the patient what they want to hear or avoid answering the question because you feel uncomfortable. At the same time you should be sensitive in your approach.

Option B: Not only is this giving the patient false information (you have no clue at this point whether it is cancer or not) it is very insensitive in its approach. Even if you had a feeling that it was likely to be cancer there are more sensitive ways to break the news. Thus Option B is not appropriate.

Option C: Although this approach may theoretically be a good idea as the patient may need some support to deal with the fact she may have cancer, this option is not appropriate. This is mainly because you are avoiding the patient's question which is likely to make her worry even more. Also by telling her that she may need a friend present to hear the news she is likely to assume the worst, which may not be the case. Thus Option C is not appropriate.

Option E: Again this approach avoids answering the patient's question. Although you may not have a definitive answer at this time, the patient is understandably worried and you need to at least try and address their concerns as best you can. In view that there are two other options (A and D) that at least attempt to address the patient's concerns, Option E is not appropriate.

Option A: This approach is honest and recognises that the patient does have a right to know that cancer is a possibility. Unlike the other options it does not avoid answering the question but gives the patient an honest answer and explains that more tests are needed to be clear of the diagnosis. Thus Option A is an appropriate and sensitive approach to take.

Option D: This option acknowledges that although the diagnosis may be cancer there are other possible diagnoses. By informing the patient of the other pathologies the shadow may represent you are trying to give them a little hope that it may not be cancer. However, by reiterating that the shadowing could also be cancer you are not falsely reassuring them that everything will be fine. Thus Option D is also appropriate and together with Option A are the most appropriate actions to the situation.

Partial Marks

You would have gained little or no marks for answering that Options B or C were appropriate. However, some of you may have felt more comfortable telling the patient that the chest clinic would be able to answer her question better after their investigations, thinking this was the safest approach (Option E). Some of you may have ranked Options A and E or possibly Options D and E as the two most appropriate actions. Although, you would be right in telling the patient that the chest clinic will be able to give her a definitive answer after their tests the patient is worried and reaching out to you for some sort of help. Although you do not have the definitive answer to her question at this time, it is far more appropriate to give her some sort of answer with the evidence and details that you have at this moment. Thus informing her that it possibly could be cancer but it is not for certain as yet or indeed informing her of the other possibilities the shadow could represent, is far more appropriate than not giving the patient any answer at all.

Question 14
Answer: 1.B 2.C 3.D 4.A 5.E

This question looks at your professional integrity and addresses the issue of patient safety. Although you may be a junior doctor, you have a duty to protect your patients even if that means informing a senior of any concerns you have with a colleague. As this is a question that involves addressing potential performance issues of another colleague we can use the approach as recommended in Chapter 2. Firstly, we need to establish if there is indeed an issue and if we have enough evidence to prove this. Secondly, we need to decide if there is a patient safety issue. In this question there is obviously an issue. We are observing the issue with our own eyes and thus we have enough evidence to feel that the Registrar is not competent. This is not hearsay. In view of this, the issue needs to be addressed and it needs to be addressed immediately as there are patient safety issues. It would not be safe to let this doctor continue if he is making serious mistakes and we need to do something about it urgently.

Options B and C: These appear to be the most appropriate actions to take out of the options we have been given. We have already stated that we need to address this issue immediately and safeguard the patients and thus we need to make this a priority. Contacting the Consultant on call allows a senior with medical experience to handle the situation. It may be that he needs to come down and review the patients seen by the Registrar to ensure that they have been correctly managed. He is also in a better position to contact medical staffing and inform them of what has happened than you are. However, after that it may be appropriate to contact medical staffing yourself as although this Registrar needs to be stopped from seeing patients you will need a replacement. Option B is therefore the most appropriate action and Option C is the 2nd most appropriate.

Option D: Confronting the Registrar in front of the patients is not ideal. It will achieve little and may upset the patients. However, although this is inappropriate it is at least trying to do something about the situation unlike the remaining two options where the Registrar is left to his own devices. At least by explaining to the Registrar how you think the case should be managed there is a possibility that the case will be managed correctly, especially if the Registrar simply does not know how to handle the case due to lack of experience. Thus Option D is the 3rd most appropriate action.

Options A and E: If we really analyse these options we can see that they have one thing in common. They both involve leaving the Registrar on the wards around the patients. Thus they are inappropriate as the patients are likely to be at risk. However, the patients are even more likely to be at risk due to inadequate cover, if you decide to walk out on your shift. Not only will they have an incompetent on call Registrar providing their care they will have no on call foundation doctor. As stated in Chapter 2, you must always ensure there is adequate cover to look after your patients at the end of your shift, to simply walk out is unprofessional and unsafe. Thus Option E is the least appropriate action, which leaves Option A as the 4th most appropriate action.

Partial mark answer
You would have scored partial marks for ranking CBDAE, i.e. calling medical staffing first before your Consultant. Those of you who did so may have felt that as it may take time to find a replacement it is better to contact medical staffing first so they can start trying to find cover. However, your immediate duty is to

ensure the safety and well-being of your patients. Medical staffing is in no position to give you any senior advice on the medical care of your patients. Also it is common courtesy to let the Consultant on call know immediately if there are any patient safety issues as ultimately he is responsible for the patients that day. Thus Option B ranks before C in the model answer.

Question 15
Answer: 1.C 2.E 3.B 4.D 5.A

This question represents a critical event and one that has put a patient at risk. When dealing with critical events there is a set approach that can be applied to most of the questions. Your first duty is to stabilise the patient and reduce the risk to the patient. You then have a duty to try and explore why the event happened and to take measures to try and ensure it does not happen again. Thus, as with most of the questions that involve patient safety issues, you should prioritise your actions which deal with the patient safety issue immediately.

Option C: In view of this Option C has to be the most appropriate action. The patient's blood pressure is low and we need to do something about this immediately. Thus you need to get a nurse to put up the fluids as soon as possible. Even if you feel that you need some further input from your Registrar, having IV fluids will not harm the patient whilst you are speaking to him, and it makes sense to do this first to try and stabilise the patient. Thus Option C is the most appropriate action.

Option E: The natural second step to take after the fluids have gone up is to speak to your Registrar for further advice. He may suggest that you increase the rate of the fluids or may come to review the patient with you. Again this is trying to deal with the immediate patient safety issue and thus Option E is the 2nd most appropriate action.

Option A: Although this too would be attempting to deal with the immediate patient safety issue, it is inappropriate as it is unsafe. We are unsure of how to set up the IV fluids and thus it is safer, and more appropriate, to ask a nurse to do it, than to do it ourselves and risk getting it wrong. In view of the fact that this could increase the risk to the patient Option A is the least appropriate answer.

We are now left with two options, both of which involve trying to get to the bottom of why this incident occurred and to try and prevent it happening again.

Options D and B: Option D involves confronting the nurse and is unlikely to achieve anything. Although a mistake was made we are unsure as to the reasons why. To belittle the nurse in front of everyone would be unprofessional. It is far more appropriate to fill in an incident form where the reasons behind why this occurred would be investigated without a fellow colleague being berated. Thus Option D is more appropriate than Option B, and are the 3rd and 4th most appropriate actions respectively.

Although, Option A was attempting to deal with the situation immediately, whereas Options D and B tried to prevent it from happening again, Option A is still the least appropriate answer. This is because it is unsafe and could place the patient in more danger, which is obviously worse than confronting the nurse, although neither of the options are ideal.

Partial mark answer

You would have scored partial marks for ranking Option E in front of Option C, (i.e. ECDBA), and calling your Registrar first. Although, you may have been worried about this patient, this should be a scenario as a foundation doctor you are trained to deal with on a basic level. IV fluids are appropriate and would have done no harm to the patient, whilst you were waiting to speak to the Registrar. You should at least try to stabilise the patient first, especially as you are not sure where your Registrar is or how long they will take to respond. Thus in the model answer Option C ranked before Option E.

Question 16
Answer: B, D and F

This question assesses your professional integrity and your willingness to be accountable for your own actions. It is based on these ethical principles but also addresses your teamworking skills. You signed the prescription and are the one who is likely to be held accountable. However, on the other hand there are probably a few other factors that contributed to this significant event. It may be that the letter was misfiled or there was poor communication between primary and secondary care. You could also argue that the nurse should have checked before giving the injection. However, this is not dealing with the issue at hand. And placing the blame on others is futile and is only likely to cause offence.

Options A and E: Here you are blaming someone else for the event. You are also being confrontational in your approach by giving someone a 'telling off' about what they should not have done. This is not the correct way of doing things. For one you were the one that signed the prescription. However, although there may be several other factors leading up to the mistake this should be dealt with in a 'blame-free' manner. In this way, no one is made to feel personally responsible for what happened. Thus to blame the nurse or the person who had filed the original letter is not appropriate at all.

Option B: Based on what has previously been said, calling a practice meeting and conducting a significant event analysis seems like a sensible action. Here the matter is dealt with in a structured way. It can be kept entirely confidential and aims at finding ways to prevent the matter from happening again rather than blaming particular individuals. Thus Option B is an appropriate action to take.

Option C: Again this is blaming somebody for what has happened and does not demonstrate good teamwork or communication skills. You may feel pressured when asked to sign a prescription quickly but to place the blame on the receptionist is not acceptable. Although, it may be sensible to have a policy where doctors are not asked to sign prescriptions without having time to check the notes, it is better that this is proposed in the practice meeting rather than you personally telling the receptionists they should not do so. Thus Option C is not appropriate.

Option D: This is an honest and sensible approach. The GMC clearly states that if an error has been made you must be honest and open with the patient and apologise promptly and explain the short term and long term impacts of what has happened. Thus if any error has occurred you must inform the patient of the error and be apologetic in doing so. Thus Option D is an appropriate action to take.

Option F: Discussing the matter with the person responsible for your training at the surgery is a wise thing to do. Not only are you informing someone senior of the event, but you are also allowing yourself to reflect on your thoughts and feelings over the incident. Naturally, you will probably be quite upset and worried over what has happened and it is important to reflect on your experience and learn from it. It is not only useful to learn from it in terms of finding ways to not be in that situation again but will also be good for your personal development. Hence Option F is an appropriate action.

Option G: Speaking to one of your junior colleagues may be helpful in having someone to empathise with what has happened but is unlikely to benefit the patient or the practice. In view of the fact you have an option to speak to your trainer instead, Option G is not the most appropriate action.

Thus actions B, D and F are the most appropriate three actions to take.

Question 17
Answer: A, B and D

This question once again represents a scenario where a patient's safety may be at risk from a significant event. As seen in previous questions, we must act immediately to ensure that the patient is well and stable. Once we have removed or dealt with the risk to the patient we can then take steps to prevent the incident from happening again. We should also always act with integrity and be honest with patients when mistakes are made and must never cover up mistakes from patients. We also have a duty to inform the patients of the consequences of any mistake we have made.

Options A and D: These are the only two options that involve taking active steps to ensure that the risk to the patient is dealt with immediately. By consulting a senior colleague immediately we are ensuring that we follow the correct procedures to ensure the patient's safety. Similarly by reviewing the medication guidelines as to what the side effects may be, we are able to spot these in the patient and also able to inform the patient of what the possible ill effect of this mild overdose may be.

Options F and G: Although you may need to inform your Consultant when you see him or bring up the error during a ward meeting, these options are not the most appropriate in view of the fact that they do not take immediate action. Thus Options F and G are not appropriate as there are other more appropriate actions that we would consider first.

Option E: Informing your ward nurse that everything is fine is dishonest and does not address the fact that the patient has been given a mild overdose. Thus this option is not appropriate at all.

Options B and C: Option B is sensible as you should be honest with the patient if a mistake has been made and inform them as soon as possible. Also, by documenting it in the patient's notes you are ensuring that anyone coming into contact with this patient knows about what has happened, and can provide the best care for the patient with this knowledge in mind.

Completing a critical incident form is also sensible in that it will try to analyse why this event happened and possibly look at ways to prevent it. However, if we are comparing these two actions, Option B is more appropriate as it involves taking more immediate action about the situation.

This leaves us with Options A, B and D as the three most appropriate actions to take.

Question 18
Answer: 1.C 2.E 3.D 4.A 5.B

This question is deliberately ambiguous and involves a delicate situation where you need to consider patient safety together with professional courtesy to your colleague. As stated in Chapter 2, when dealing with possible conduct issues in colleagues, it is important to decide whether there is an issue that indeed needs to be addressed and whether you have conclusive evidence. However as we have discussed previously, if there is or potentially could be a patient safety issue then you must not ignore the situation.

Although we have no conclusive evidence that the Consultant has or intended to have any alcohol, as patients could be at potential risk if he is drinking on the job, we cannot ignore the situation. However, we must remember that we have no real evidence at this point in time that he has done anything wrong and should not be overly confrontational and assume the worst.

Options A and B: In view of this these two options are obviously inappropriate. Option B we do nothing at all, assuming it is completely innocent and Option A we assume the worst and overreact by informing the GMC. Informing the GMC is extreme and by not giving your Consultant a chance to respond is unfair but, it is better than doing nothing. This is simply because by doing nothing patients could be at risk and this is never acceptable. Thus Option B is the least appropriate action and Option A is the 2nd least appropriate action.

Option C: Conversely, the most appropriate action is to at least allow the Consultant a chance to explain himself. By asking your Consultant the circumstances under which he placed the bottle of alcohol in the drawer you are giving him a chance to respond and seeing whether there is a completely logical explanation before taking the matter further. Thus Option C is the most appropriate action.

Option D: This option is unlikely to be helpful. By asking his secretary if she has noticed anything, you are not only assuming the worst, but could be seen as starting rumour and gossip. She may also inform the Consultant of your questioning which may cause offence, especially as you did not come and speak to him first. This approach is also unlikely to provide you with any hard evidence of wrong doing and is likely to just cause trouble. However, it is better than doing nothing at all because patients could be at risk and at least it attempts to address the issue. This option is also better than assuming the worst and informing the GMC. This is because the consequences of discussing it with the secretary are likely to be less than the consequences of informing the GMC, especially if there is an innocent explanation.

Option E: In this option you inform your Consultant of your concerns and advise him to see his GP. This is also assuming the worst based on little information and may cause offence. However, at least by speaking directly to your Consultant and not involving anyone else you cannot be accused of gossiping. Also, it involves suggesting a way to help the situation should there be one, whereas asking his secretary questions does not really solve any potential problem. Therefore Option E is more appropriate than Option D and Option E ranks as the 2nd most appropriate action. Therefore leaving Option D as the 3rd most appropriate action.

Partial mark answer
There is not a partial mark answer to this question that would score a high number of marks. Some of you however, may have ranked Option D in front of Option E choosing to question his secretary before informing the Consultant you are concerned. Although you may feel rather uncomfortable advising the Consultant to see his GP with very little evidence at all, it is important to remember that in both options you are assuming the worst and jumping to conclusions. However, it is better in general to try and deal with the matter as locally as possible and not gossip or involve other staff unnecessarily. As the secretary has no authority to do anything about the Consultant it makes little sense involving her. If you are going to jump to a conclusion that may be false, it is better to limit this to just between you and the Consultant rather than to spread this information to other staff and possibly around the hospital.

Question 19
Answer: B, C and F
This is a difficult situation which assesses your sensitivity, communication skills and your relationships with colleagues. A complaint made about your fellow colleague who is at the same level as you could make you feel rather uncomfortable especially when the responsibility is left to you to sort the matter out.

The first thing you need to think about is whether there is an issue at hand. Although, there is no specific dress code for doctors we have a responsibility to maintain trust in the profession and dress appropriately. Thus wearing very short clothing could potentially offend patients. As such, this could be a more serious issue especially if patients have complained. Although, you may not feel comfortable dealing with the situation the nurse may not have wanted to get any senior involved, and may have just asked you to have an informal chat with your colleague rather than making it a formal matter. Thus, although you may feel uncomfortable you should bear this in mind before involving others.

Option C: In view of what has been said this seems like the most sensible option. Here you speak informally to your colleague informing her of what has been said before getting anyone more senior involved. This has the benefit of not embarrassing your colleague any further or causing her unnecessary concern by involving a consultant. It also gives her the opportunity to rectify the situation before it escalates any further. Thus Option C is an appropriate action to take.

Option A: Although with this approach you are suggesting she change her attire. This may not be successful as you are not providing a reason why, because in your mind you do not want to cause offence. You may not be involving seniors but by dropping hints that she should dress differently, you are not directly addressing the situation as asked to by a fellow colleague. It may also come across that it is your personal opinion that she is dressed incorrectly, as you have not told her what has been discussed, resulting in personal conflict. Thus Option A is not appropriate.

Option G: Although again this option does not involve a senior, it is creating gossip and is not appropriate. Discussing the complaint in the mess with other doctors who have nothing to do with the situation is unlikely to benefit your colleague or help you to decide what to do, and is likely to just start rumours. Thus Option G is not appropriate.

Option D: Although you may feel that there is not an issue with your colleague's dress sense, to tell the nurse you will deal with the matter and then not addressing it at all, is being dishonest. Although you may not feel it is your role to mention it to your colleague, you cannot ignore what has been said. If you do not tell your colleague what has been said and she continues to dress the same way, the situation may escalate further resulting in the Consultant and other seniors becoming involved when it could have been addressed sooner. Thus Option D is not appropriate.

Option E: This option is not ideal as medical personnel are not the best people to deal with this type of scenario. If you are going to involve a senior, in view of the other options, it would be more appropriate to involve your Registrar who actually knows the person at hand. It would not be fair to your colleague to involve medical personnel when the situation could be dealt with more locally, e.g. by your Registrar.

Option F: Although, ideally you may want to try and deal with this situation locally without involving your seniors, it is a difficult situation. Therefore it may be sensible to discuss it with your Registrar yourself and ask them to handle the situation if you feel uncomfortable. Although, this may seem like shirking responsibility it is a far better option that informing other colleagues that have nothing to do with the matter or informing medical personnel who will probably not want to get involved and go to your Consultant anyway. It is also much better than dealing with a situation you feel uncomfortable with and causing more offence to your colleague by dealing with it incorrectly. Thus Option F is appropriate in view of the other options.

Option B: Similarly it may also be sensible therefore to ask the nurse to speak to your colleague themselves or your Registrar, if you really feel uncomfortable talking to your colleague yourself. Although, this again may feel like you are shirking responsibility it is better to be honest with the nurse and tell her you are not comfortable dealing with the situation than to ignore it or deal with it incorrectly. Thus Option B is appropriate in view of the other options.

Thus Options B, C and F are the most appropriate actions to take.

Question 20
Answer: B and D
This question represents a common scenario in general practice. It addresses your empathy and communication skills as well as your principles on good prescribing. It is quite easy to become intimidated when patients are overly demanding and give in to their demands. However, we must also remember that we have a duty to do what is best for our patients and prescribe correctly. If we prescribe antibiotics inappropriately we may be contributing to problems with resistance. Also, although prescribing antibiotics when warranted can cause side effects, at least we could argue that the benefits outweigh the risks. However, it is hard to argue giving a medication that possibly has side effects when there is no indication for that medication at all. On the other hand, we do have a stressed single mother with four

children. One can empathise that having a sick child at this time must be very demanding for her and we do have a duty to be sympathetic to this.

Option A: Although this may be in the mother's best interests it is the child we are treating here. We have a duty to prescribe 'appropriately and in the patient's best interests' in accordance with the GMC and thus to simply give the child antibiotics because you do not wish to argue with the mother is irresponsible. It may be that after a long discussion with the mother you decide to give or not give the antibiotic for whatever reason, but you should at least attempt to explain your reasoning to the mother. She may just require a more detailed explanation as to why the antibiotics are not appropriate. Thus to simply give in to the demanding mother without even an attempt to resolve the situation is not appropriate.

Option B: This seems like a more sensible idea. Here we empathise with the fact that she is a single mother and must be stressed. This is likely to calm the mother and show her that we understand her point of view. By pointing out the side effects of the antibiotics, we are giving her both the risks and benefits of the treatment. It may be that after showing some sympathy and explaining to her properly why antibiotics are not necessary that she agrees to follow our advice. Thus Option B is an appropriate action to take.

Option C: Although we are well within our rights to decline the mother's request for antibiotics, if we do not deem it to be in the best interest of the child, we should show some empathy. To simply refuse the mother without even listening to her concerns or attempting to explain again why they are not necessary is not the best course of action. So although not giving the antibiotics may be appropriate, the wording of the question may indicate that there may be other suitable options.

Option E: Although patients are entitled to a second opinion if they wish, this action is really passing the demanding mother onto one of our colleagues. Our colleague is likely to feel the same way as us and thus it is likely to be counterproductive in this situation. As the mother is stressed and is finding it difficult to manage her time, there may be more suitable options than asking her to rebook with another colleague which is likely to aggravate her more.

Option D: Here you offer her a delayed prescription, where if the child becomes worse she can take it to the pharmacy without the need to see a doctor. This can often be a suitable compromise as some mother's feel comforted by the fact they have this safety net. Although we do run the risk that the mother may just get the antibiotics immediately, it is at least trying to establish some sort of compromise and will negate the need for the mother to book another appointment with your colleague saving both time and money. Thus Option D is appropriate and is more appropriate than Option E.

This leaves us with Options B and D as the two most appropriate actions.

Question 21
Answer: C and E

This question is designed to test your ability to problem solve as well as your professional and personal integrity. There are three issues in this question. One is your duty of care to your patients and the fact that they need a refreshed doctor who has not stayed up all night. The second issue is your duty to provide accurate data in your clinical audit. The third and final issue is your duty to act with honesty and integrity and therefore not lie to others including your supervisor.

Option A: This is plainly unsafe. It is 3am and you need to be up in a few hours. Although you have a duty to provide your supervisor with the data it would not be acceptable to put your patients at risk in order to complete the data. Also you are unlikely to be able to concentrate on the audit and may make your data prone to errors. Thus Option A is inappropriate as it may put patients at risk and there are other options which are far more appropriate.

Options B and D: Both these options involve being dishonest. In Option B you forge the data which would be dishonest. As audits are designed to evaluate whether you are providing good standards of care, to have incorrect data may actually affect the whole outcome of your audit and is not appropriate. You only have to present the raw data tomorrow and not the final audit, thus there is plenty of time to look through the ten remaining notes, albeit not tonight. With Option D you are now lying to your supervisor because you are perhaps too cowardly to tell him the truth. Although this may grant you a reprieve it is never best practice to lie and there are other more appropriate options. Thus Options B and D are not appropriate.

Option C: This seems like a sensible option. You only have to submit the raw data to your supervisor and although you should have been more prepared they are likely to not be too upset as you only have a few more notes to look through. This approach shows that you are being honest and taking responsibility for the fact that you did not complete your task on time, instead of lying and finding ways to avoid the situation. It will also negate the need for you to stay up exhausted and possibly put patients at risk the following day. Thus Option C is appropriate.

Option E: Although trying to complete the data the following day is not ideal it is more appropriate than the other options. As the question states that it will take you about an hour to look through the notes it is feasible to attempt to complete this the next day during a break. Even if you cannot look through all the notes you may be able to get most of it done, so that if you do need to admit to your supervisor that you haven't completed everything, you can reassure him that you only have a couple of patient notes to look through. Although it is possible that you may not have time to complete the data it is at least worth a try. This is obviously better than being dishonest or putting patients at risk by staying up late and turning up for work exhausted. Thus Option E is an appropriate action to take.

This makes Options C and E the two most appropriate actions to take.

Question 22
Answer: 1.E 2.D 3.B 4.C 5.A

This question assesses how we work with colleagues and our empathy and sensitivity. Although we may be keen to help a colleague out on occasions, this scenario represents one where a colleague is not pulling their weight. It could have implications on patient safety if, for example, there was an emergency that required your colleague's presence. As it involves a potential patient safety issue it is not one that you can ignore. However, we do need to be sympathetic and courteous to our colleague, and deal with the situation in an appropriate manner.

Option A: Based on the fact that patient safety could potentially be compromised by the lack of your colleague's presence, Option A is the least appropriate action as it involves ignoring the situation.

Option E: This is obviously the most appropriate action as you are dealing with the matter by being sensitive and enquiring into the reasons behind your colleague's behaviour. Your colleague may have childcare or other issues that mean she needs to leave early. Although this does not make her behaviour acceptable it may be something that you can deal with together without involving seniors.

Option D: This option also involves addressing the issue directly with your colleague unlike the other two available options (B and C) where you involve others. Although, it is ideal to discuss the matter with your colleague before approaching others, warning your colleague about her behaviour does not show much sensitivity or empathy at all. This approach may also be deemed confrontational and is not ideal. However, at least you give her the chance to respond to your concerns and try to amend the situation before involving your seniors. Thus Option D is more appropriate than Option B or C and is the 2nd most appropriate action.

Options B and C: These options involve informing others of the situation at hand. Option B where you go directly to your Consultant seems a bit drastic and without enquiring into the reasons behind your colleague leaving early seems a bit harsh. However, to go behind your colleague's back (Option C) and discuss your concerns with the whole ward staff and her friends is even more inappropriate as you may be seen as gossiping. By discussing it with the staff, you are only establishing opinions and rumours, and are not really addressing the issue. Also, if your colleague does genuinely have a good reason for leaving early, by bringing it to the whole ward's attention you have already given the ward a bad impression of your colleague. Therefore although they are both inappropriate Option B is more appropriate than Option C due to the fact that you are actually dealing with the matter and not simply spreading rumours. Thus Option B is the 3rd most appropriate action and Option C the 4th.

Partial marks
Had you ranked Option B before Options E and D (i.e. BEDCA), with you feeling more comfortable to inform the Consultant than to confront your colleague you would have scored partial marks. Confronting a colleague is not ideal and is not something that everyone feels able to do. However, going straight to the Consultant without even giving your colleague a chance to remedy the situation or respond is a bit severe. Also involving the consultant in such a simple matter may not be logical or ideal. It may perhaps be more appropriate to ask your Registrar or her educational supervisor to deal with such a matter, where it may be dealt with more informally.

Question 23
Answer: 1.D 2.A 3.C 4.E 5.B
Although we all have a responsibility to behave professionally and maintain trust in the profession we are all entitled to let our hair down after hours and have personal lives! However, if a colleague's conduct in their personal life

posed a risk to a patient e.g. smoking marijuana in their personal time, then we would have a duty to address it. Therefore when addressing this question we need to look at the basic rules discussed in Chapter 2 on 'whistle blowing'; i.e. is there an issue at hand, do we have enough evidence and is there a patient safety issue, as this cannot be ignored.

If we analyse this situation based on these rules, there really isn't an issue at hand. It is a staff party, there are no patients present and no harm has been done. There certainly isn't a patient safety issue and thus we can ignore what has been heard. Therefore, to penalise the nurses for a bit of drunken banter seems a bit over the top and is likely to damage your relationship with them.

Option D: Thus the appropriate answer to this question is to do nothing. There is not an issue that needs to be addressed at all. Thus Option D is the most appropriate action.

Based on this all the remaining options are inappropriate but we still need to prioritise them. As we have determined that we should not do anything in this situation, we need to rank the other answers based on the severity of the action.

Option B: Out of the actions provided, this seems the most severe in that it involves going to the most senior person. As we have discussed in Chapter 2, this is not appropriate and you should always try and address the matter locally before progressing up the hierarchy. It also seems pointless as your Consultant has little to do with the training of the nursing staff. Thus Option B is the least appropriate option.

Options A and C: It would seem more sensible to discuss the issue with the nurses themselves instead of involving anyone else. Thus it would be more appropriate to choose a tactful time to discuss the matter than confronting the nurses directly. Thus Option A is the 2nd most appropriate action (after Option D) and is more appropriate than Option C as it involves being more tactful. Option C although confrontational, is better than involving anyone more senior in this trivial matter. Thus Option C is the 3rd most appropriate option.

Option E: This describes involving a senior and therefore ranks after Options A and C. As it involves informing someone lower down the hierarchy than the Consultant, and at least someone who is involved with the training of the nursing staff, it ranks higher than Option B. Therefore Option E is the 4th most appropriate action.

Partial mark answer

Some of you may have ranked confronting the nursing staff as the least appropriate action (i.e. DAEBC). Although confronting your colleagues is never ideal, we have to look at it in view of the remaining options. In this case where there really is not an issue at hand it would be far more unsuitable to involve seniors as this is likely to lead to a more adverse outcome than if you confront the nurses themselves. This would have been different perhaps if there really was an issue, such as a patient safety issue, when it would have been more beneficial to involve someone to address the issue than to confront the nurses which would achieve nothing. However, in this scenario there is not an issue, and the situation could be rapidly eliminated by voicing your opinions to the nurses directly. Although this may cause offence it is unlikely to cause as much offence as involving seniors in such a trivial matter. Therefore although you would score partial marks for ranking Option C last it is not the model answer.

Question 24
Answer: 1.C 2.B 3.A 4.D

This question revolves around confidentiality issues in minors and not only assesses your awareness of the guidelines but your sensitivity and communication skills. Minors have the same confidentiality rights as those of adults, and you should attempt to maintain confidentiality at all times. The exceptions where you are allowed to break confidentiality for adults are essentially the same in children. However, when dealing with children in particular, you may have a child protection issue where you need to break confidentiality or the child may not be mature enough to consent. In the latter case you may need to inform their parents if you feel their knowledge is necessary to provide proper care for the child.

In this scenario, we are told that the child is mature and intelligent and thus is likely to be able to consent for herself. Although we are told she has a boyfriend we are not given any indication that there is any child protection issue, or that there is anything underhand going on. Indeed many 14 year olds these days have boyfriends! Thus we have no grounds to breach her confidentiality by informing her mother about her boyfriend.

Options A and D: In view of what has been said these options are the least appropriate. To assume that as she is a little down that something untoward has gone on with the boyfriend is reading too much into the situation. Thus we have no real reason to go and break her confidentiality and tell her mother. We have even less reason to go and inform social services. We have no indication from the information provided that there is a child protection issue here, nor can we assume bad parenting because a 14 year old is in a relationship. That view would be judgemental and in this day and age a little outdated. However, if we were going to go and break her confidentiality it would be more appropriate to tell her mother than social services as we have little evidence that there are any child protection issues going on. Thus Option D is even less appropriate than Option A as it involves taking more drastic measures. This leaves Option D as the least appropriate action and Option A as the 2nd least appropriate action.

We are now left with two options which both involve respecting the patient's confidentiality which would be the correct stance to take in this case. We have stated that we have no evidence of any concerns in this situation so it would be correct to respect the patient's right to confidentiality. We now have to prioritise between these two appropriate options.

Options B and C: In Option C we respect the patient's right to confidentiality but also recognise the fact that her mother is anxious. Although we cannot force her to confide in her mother, by suggesting she speaks to her mother we are at least trying to establish some communication between them. She is likely to need some support through this time and her mother may be more understanding if she knows what is going on. We cannot however force her to do this and if she refuses we should respect her wishes. With Option B we simply just tell the mother that we cannot divulge any information. Although we are correct in saying so it seems more helpful to at least suggest to the teenager that she involves her mother. If she then declined we could then resort to Option B. Thus Option C is more appropriate than Option B and thus Option C is the most appropriate option. This leaves Option B ranking as the 2nd most appropriate action to take.

Partial mark answer

You would have scored partial marks for ranking Option B in front of Option C (i.e. BCAD). However, it is more logical to talk to the patient and suggest she informs her mother, well before you need to tell the mother you cannot reveal anything. By doing this at least you give the daughter a chance to think about whether to inform her mother. This may alleviate the need for you to be in the position where you tell the mother that you cannot tell her what has been discussed with her daughter.

Question 25
Answer: C and E

This scenario looks at the issue of confidentiality once again. Although the patient is well within her rights to not want you to reveal to anyone that her partner is abusing her, the situation is entirely different if the children are at risk. As stated when discussing confidentially and child protection issues in Chapter 2, you are allowed to break confidentiality if you feel a child may be at risk. Here we have a clear cut case where a child was actually hit by her violent partner and thus we cannot ignore it. We have a duty to protect those children even if it means breaking the patient's confidentiality.

Option A: In view of this Option A is inappropriate. By not revealing this situation to social services we will be putting these children at risk. Thus we have a duty to protect them and must not simply keep quiet because their mother wants us to.

Option B: Although the police may need to be involved down the line, calling the police immediately is unlikely to help. We are breaking confidentiality in order to protect the children, not the mother. The mother does not wish the police to be involved and involving them at this stage is unlikely to protect the children immediately, and therefore we would have little reason to break her confidentiality and call them. If anything, the police would contact social services about the children and it makes more sense to contact them instead first. Had the injuries to either the children or the mother been severe this may have been appropriate. However, with the information we have there are more appropriate actions to take.

Option C: Social services are likely to be helpful in this situation. They can not only give us advice but arrange for this matter to be taken further and to ensure the children are safe and protected. They will not necessarily take the children away but will try to make sure the children are safe and offer any support they can. You should however ask for the patient's permission to break confidentiality, even if the mother did not give her consent, you should still contact social services to protect the children. Ideally, you should inform the mother of your need to do so. Thus Option C is appropriate.

Option D: Contacting her partner is unlikely to be helpful. Here you are breaching her confidentiality once again. However, you could not justify that you needed to break her confidentiality here to protect either the children or her in this circumstance. By contacting her partner and informing him that she has told you of what has happened you risk angering him further, and possibly placing them more at risk. Thus Option D is not appropriate.

Option E: Although this does not deal with any child protection issues immediately, it may help her to leave her husband should she choose to do so. Although, the needs of the child are paramount we should also consider the mother here and try to help and support her. Even though she currently wishes to stay in the relationship, we should at least inform her of her other options. This is likely to help her more than calling the police against her wishes. Thus Option E is appropriate.

This leaves us with Options C and E as the two most appropriate actions to take.

Partial Marks

You would have scored partial marks for ranking Options B and C as the most appropriate actions. Some of you may have felt it more beneficial to call the police immediately than to give the mother domestic violence information. Although this would be dealing with the situation you need to look at your reasons for calling the police. You would be doing it to protect the children and as such social services would be a much better option to ensure the children's safety. Also calling the police would not protect the mother as she may not wish to press any charges, and as social services would be able to deal with the children safety issue it seems more reasonable to offer the mother some sort of support. The police would be more help in a situation where either the patient or her children are in immediate danger and her partner needs to be removed. However, you would not be marked down too severely had you chosen to call the police.

Question 26
Answer: 1.D 2.C 3.A 4.B 5.E

This question looks at the issue of confidentiality versus patient safety. Here you have an adult who has been a victim of domestic violence. However, she does not wish to take this matter further and thus you need to decide whether you will respect that or break her confidentiality. You should always try to respect the patient's right to confidentiality; however, it can be broken in a few situations. We may be entitled to break confidentiality if we could prove that the benefit to the individual outweighed the disadvantages of keeping the information confidential. This may be the case if we needed to break confidentiality to immediately protect her from serious harm or death. Although, this may be the case if her injuries were severe, it is difficult to argue that this is the case with a few old bruises.

However, this does not mean that you cannot advise the patient of their options including advice on women's refuges or domestic abuse help lines. This is explaining how she could obtain help and support should she need it. This is not the same as telling the patient to leave her husband and we should not be judgemental or try to influence the patient in any way.

Option E: This is the least appropriate answer. Here we break the patient's confidentiality against her wishes but also to her partner. We have stated already that we should respect her confidentiality unless we felt that we needed to break confidentiality to protect her from death or serious harm. However, by breaking her confidentiality to her partner we may be putting her at more risk and therefore cannot justify this approach. Thus Option E is the least appropriate action as it involves both breaking her confidentiality and putting her at risk.

Option D: Although she may not want to take the matter further and involve the police she has revealed the situation to you and this may be a cry for help. She may be scared and hence the reason why she does not wish to contact the police. You should not try to influence her in any way but do have a duty to offer her help and support. It seems sensible to inform her of her options and let her decide what she feels is best for her. Thus Option D is the most appropriate action.

Option C: This again appears to be a sensible action. She may change her mind in the future and although we should always keep accurate notes, it may be important to record extra detail in this consultation in case it does go to court. You may be required to provide evidence with regards to her injuries and it is important to make sure you have documented these. It is however, not directly helping the patient with the situation at hand and although it is appropriate ranks as the 2nd most appropriate action behind Option D.

Options A and B: You are now left with two options. Either respect her wishes and do nothing or call the police. As we have already said that we would have little grounds in this case to break her confidentiality we cannot justify at this stage going to the police behind her back. Thus Option A ranks as the 3rd most appropriate action leaving Option B as the 4th most appropriate action.

Although with both Options B and E her confidentiality is broken, Option E involves putting her at increased risk of harm and remains the least appropriate action to take.

Partial Marks

You would have scored partial marks for ranking Option C in front of Option D, i.e. documenting everything clearly before explaining to the patient her options. This may be logical in that you obviously need to document everything she states about the abuse clearly and any injuries you note, and thus it may be a logical place to start. However, as stated several times you should always try to select actions that deal with the issue at hand immediately. It is therefore better to choose informing the patient about her rights and her options as your most appropriate action as documenting everything clearly does not help the patient with the immediate situation.

Question 27
Answer: 1.C 2.D 3.A 4.B 5.E

This is a question that checks your professional integrity, organisation and planning as well as your problem solving ability. The GMC provides clear guidance on arranging cover:

> 'You must be satisfied that, when you are off duty, suitable arrangements have been made for your patients' medical care. These arrangements should include effective handover procedures, involving clear communication with healthcare colleagues'.

Option C: The most appropriate action is obviously to find out what has happened to your colleague as this will determine what you need to do next. Your colleague may simply be five minutes away and you can therefore wait for him or he may actually have called in sick in which case you may need to make other arrangements. Thus Option C is the most appropriate answer.

Option E: The other options involve various methods of handover or staying until your colleague or cover arrives. As you have just completed a night shift you are unlikely to be in any fit state to carry on working a day shift as well. You are also needed for another night shift later and to stay on during the day would be compromising patient safety. You have no idea where your colleague is or when cover will arrive so to stay until this happens is not in the best interest of patient safety. Thus Option E is the least appropriate action.

You are now left with three handover options: personally to your Registrar or Consultant or to leave a detailed list of the jobs. As just discussed the GMC has stated that we have a clear responsibility to have effective handover procedures which would include handing over appropriately and to the correct person.

Options A and D: From the remaining actions it is more appropriate to hand over to someone personally than to leave a list in an office. You are likely to be able to give a more effective handover by communicating to someone directly than by simply writing it down as a list. Out of the two options between whom to hand over to, it is more appropriate to hand over to the day Registrar. This is mainly because they will be dealing with the patients during the day and will be working directly with your colleague when he arrives or the replacement does. The Consultant on the other hand is unlikely to be on the ward for the rest of the day and is unlikely to have any dealings with the day foundation doctor at all. Thus Option D is more appropriate than Option A, however both are less appropriate than Option C. This means that Option D is the 2nd most appropriate action whereas Option A is the 3rd most appropriate action to take.

Option B: Leaving a list of jobs is obviously not ideal as it will not be as effective as verbally communicating to the day foundation doctor. Also you cannot guarantee that they will get the handover list although you are taking steps to ensure this happens by putting it in a safe place and letting others know it is there. It is however, slightly better and safer for the patients than working part or all of a day shift when you have just completed a night shift. Thus Option B is the second least appropriate action and ranks 4th.

Partial Marks
There is not really a partial mark answer for this question that would score high marks. However, there may be some of you who would have volunteered to stay on until someone arrives to take over and thus may have ranked Option E differently. Although, this may be seen as the noble thing to do, you have no idea when someone will be coming to relieve you of your duties and it is not safe to patients for you to continue a shift when you are exhausted. It would have been different however, if your colleague was 30 minutes away and you decided to stay on for a short period.

Question 28
Answer: 1.C 2.D 3.A 4.B 5.E
This question assesses your organisational skills and how you manage your time and others. The dilemma in this scenario is that of achieving a work/life balance. You are late for an important family dinner however you do have a responsibility to ensure that when you leave your shift that your patients are adequately cared for. The fact that you have forgotten to write up the routine IV fluids for the patient does not mean that it is necessarily your job to go back and write up the fluids. However, it is your duty to ensure that the necessary

arrangements have been made to ensure your patients are cared for. As you cannot get through to the on call foundation doctor you need to try and make other arrangements.

Option E: To do nothing is not an option. Although you have a right to try and organise something so that you do not miss your dinner it is your responsibility to ensure that the fluids get written up by someone. You are the one who is aware of the fact that the patient needs to be continued on IV fluids and that they have not been written up. It is not the nurses' responsibility to figure out that the fluids have run out and need to be replaced. This is passing the responsibility to another colleague and is both unsafe for the patient and unprofessional. Thus Option E has to be the least appropriate action as it involves a possible breach in patient safety and poor teamwork and communication.

Option B: We have already stated that although we have forgotten to write up the fluids, it is our job to ensure it is handed over to someone else and not necessarily our job to miss our dinner and do it ourselves. This may have been an option if we could genuinely not get anyone else to do the job for us. However, in view of the fact that there are other options where we can manage to get the fluids written up by another colleague and still attend our dinner, Option B is not appropriate. Being late for our dinner however is more appropriate than doing nothing and possibly risking the safety of the patient. Thus Option B is the 2nd least appropriate action and ranks 4th.

We are now left with three options: two of which involve trying to deal with the situation immediately and the third option involves dealing with the matter later. When dealing with any issue that may involve patient safety you must prioritise actions that deal with the matter immediately.

Options C and D: These options both involve trying to deal with the matter immediately. Option C seems more sensible as at least then when you hand over directly to another doctor you can be sure the matter will be taken care of. It is also preferable to asking a nurse to bleep the on call doctor. Calling the ward however would also be an option if you could not contact the SHO. By contacting the senior nurse in charge you are making her aware of the fact that the patient needs to be continued on fluids and this could be handed over to all the nurses. Then once the fluids had run out the nurses on the ward would be aware that they would need to contact the on call doctor. Thus Option C is the most appropriate action and Option D is the 2nd most appropriate action.

Option A: This option is prioritised after Options C and D as it involves delaying dealing with the matter. However, at least by trying to contact the on call doctor, albeit later, you are dealing with the issue unlike Option E where you do nothing. It may be that the foundation doctor is busy at the moment and if you call later you will be able to get through to them. As it is only routine IV fluids that the patient needs, as opposed to emergency fluids to raise their blood pressure for example, there is no immediate rush. Thus it would be safe to try and contact the on call doctor later. Thus option A is the 3rd most appropriate action to take.

Partial Mark Answer

There are several partial mark variants to this question. Most of them involve the ranking of Option B (i.e. going back to the hospital). Thus you would score marks for ranking Option B perhaps as your first option (i.e. BCDAE) or as your 2nd option (if you were not able to get through to the SHO either) or even your 3rd option. However, you must remember that although this would show a great deal of commitment to work, the examiners are looking for people who can delegate and demonstrate a work/life balance. Thus although you may feel less worried to perhaps go straight back to work and do it yourself rather than ask the SHO or inform the nurses to keep trying the on call doctor, this does not show any ability to delegate. Thus you would score partial marks for placing Option B in several different places, with the exception of the least appropriate action, as it should be obvious that to do nothing is the least appropriate.

Question 29
Answer: 1.D 2.C 3.E 4.A 5.B

This scenario is one involving child protection and assesses your professional integrity and your ability to safeguard your patients. In this scenario we have a mother of an asthmatic patient who should have really ensured that he has his inhalers. However, more worryingly she did not call an ambulance when he went blue and stopped breathing. She does not seem to have any real reason for not doing so and to say that you did not want to wake up your other children when one of your children could have possibly come to harm is not acceptable. Although it may simply be lack of education that caused her to do this we do have a duty to investigate this matter further. There could possibly be a child protection issue at hand and thus we must not ignore it.

Option B: In view of this Option B is not an appropriate action. Although it is true that we should not judge our patients, and the mother may have been very stressed or perhaps did not recognise the severity of how ill her child was, to simply ignore the situation is not an option. The needs of the child are paramount, and you have a duty to investigate this matter further. Thus Option B is the least appropriate action.

Option A: Option A is similar to Option B in that you are not really addressing the issue. You are not investigating the matter by telling the mother off at all. This approach will not help you to find out whether there indeed is a child protection issue at hand and is likely to just make the mother defensive. It will also not ensure the future safety of this child. Also it shows lack of courtesy and sensitivity for the mother. Although she may need help in parenting, her child is currently unwell and to reprimand her at this time is completely insensitive. Thus Option A is the 2nd least appropriate action.

In the remaining three options you acknowledge that there may be a child protection issue and these options should therefore be prioritised. As we have mentioned before you should always aim to prioritise options that deal with the matter at hand immediately.

Options C and D: Both options involve addressing the issue immediately and protecting the child and should be your top two priorities.

Option D: This option seems sensible as you are in a hospital environment and can therefore gain some advice from someone trained in these matters. If the paediatrician felt there was indeed an issue they could then coordinate the necessary people to investigate the matter further. As a foundation doctor you may feel out of your depth calling social services immediately (Option C) when you have little information on the case. Thus Option D is more appropriate than Option C. This makes Option D the most appropriate action, with Option C being the 2nd most appropriate action.

Option E: As this child may be at risk you do have a duty to do something about the situation now. Thus although by informing the GP you will address the situation at some point it does not protect the child immediately. If the child is discharged from the hospital without any investigation he may be at risk. It is also unprofessional to pass the buck to the GP when you are the one who is seeing the child and has the immediate concern. Although the GP may need to be contacted to gain some more information and insight into the case, you cannot simply write to the GP and hope the matter gets dealt with. It does however, at least address the situation more than shouting at the mother. Thus Option E is the 3rd most appropriate action.

Partial Mark Answer

You would score partial marks for ranking Option C in front of Option D (i.e. CDEAB). This is because you have realised that the most appropriate action is to deal with this matter immediately. Although some of you would have preferred to call social services first, this may be a different approach but is still safeguarding the child. However, as we are meant to be answering this from the perspective of a FY2 doctor, it is far more appropriate to contact the necessary senior who can then follow the child protection protocol. In fact most of the child protection protocols in hospital involve contacting the paediatrician or named child protection lead before contacting social services. Thus in the model answer Option D ideally comes before Option C.

Question 30
Answer: C, D and F

This scenario probably represents one that is close to your heart! You all remember being medical students and panicking as exams are approaching and feeling ill-prepared. In this scenario it may truly be the case that the teaching he is receiving is inadequate. However, it may also be the case that he is over-reacting. In general practice anything can come through the door, thus it may simply be that there has not been many clinical signs to see, and not that his trainer has been neglectful. Thus we should not assume the worst about our colleague and keep a level head. At the same time we should also respect how the medical student feels and try to be helpful where possible.

At this moment in time, we cannot be sure that there is an issue in the level of teaching the medical student has received. We do however know that he feels he is lacking in experience of seeing patients with clinical signs. Thus it makes sense to try and do something about this in order to help the medical student in preparation for his exams.

Option D: In view of this Option D appears appropriate. Here we are not making any assumptions about the level of his teaching but are trying to address the issue. Through having a friendly chat with all the doctors in the practice and asking them to call the student in if they have any patients with good signs you are maximising the chances that the medical student will gain the experience they require. As you are doing this informally you are not going to cause any offence to anyone and the medical student is likely to feel more comfortable than if you went telling all your colleagues that he was complaining. Whether we reveal the exact details of the conversation to anyone or not, the whole point is to try and help the medical student gain his experience, thus Option D seems like a sensible option to take.

Options B and E: These options are similar in that you make the assumption that it is the practice's fault that he has not seen many patients and advise him to contact his medical school. This seems rather drastic especially as you have no evidence that there has been any wrong doing by his trainer. As previously stated, it may simply be that the patients coming through the door have not had many clinical signs and nothing to do with a lack of teaching. By telling him to contact the medical school you are now putting the practice in an unfair position and not being fair to your colleagues. Option B is also unlikely to help the medical student pass his exam, as telling the medical school about his lack of teaching after he has left the attachment will be far too late for him. Although Option E may address this matter immediately, it seems slightly drastic and there are other options that may be more suitable. Thus Options B and E are inappropriate.

Option C: This seems like a more sensible action to take rather than informing the medical school. It may be that his trainer is unaware of how he feels and can do something to remedy the situation. Thus by advising him to explain his concerns to his trainer you are trying to do something about the situation but are also being fair to your colleague. At least then his trainer has a chance to address the matter without the medical school becoming involved. Obviously, if your colleague did not address the matter you may have to advise the student to contact his medical school, however you should at least give your colleague an opportunity to remedy the situation. Thus Option C is an appropriate action to take.

Option G: Option C is distinctively different to Option G where we overreact making the assumption that our colleague has not been teaching the medical student. We have already stated that there may be a perfectly reasonable explanation for why the medical student feels ill-prepared with regard to clinical signs and it may even be that the medical student is panicking or over-reacting. Although we may wish to help this medical student out it would be unfair to go in and immediately reprimand our colleague and does not show good communication or teamworking skills. Thus Option G is inappropriate. However, had the question stated that we have a quiet chat with our colleague informing them of the medical student's concerns; it may have been an appropriate action to take.

Option A: Although it may simply be that the medical student is panicking it would not be appropriate to just ignore his concerns. Although he may very well pass with his current knowledge we cannot say that for sure and we should at least try and address his concerns. Thus Option A is not an appropriate action to take and there are other options that involve helping the medical student that should be prioritised first.

Option F: This option would involve giving the medical student some sort of support through this difficult time. Being a foundation doctor who has recently completed medical school not too long ago you are probably in the best position to understand his concerns. Thus it would be perfectly appropriate to help him out and offer to call him in should you see any patients with good clinical signs. Although you may not have any formal teaching experience this is likely to be more beneficial than ignoring his concerns or telling him to contact the medical school after his attachment. It also negates the need to put your colleague in an unfair position by advising the student to contact the medical school about his lack of teaching or reprimanding your colleague with very little evidence. Thus Option F is an appropriate action to take.

Options C, D and F are the three most appropriate actions to take.

Question 31
Answer: B, D and F

This question represents a dilemma where we have to balance our duty of care to our patients with our relationships with colleagues. We may feel sympathetic to our colleague who seems to have had too much to drink at the mess party, however, we should not make light of the situation. Not only may our colleague be unsafe around patients due to his judgement being impaired, if he gets caught smelling of alcohol by either patients or a senior he may get into serious trouble. Thus we must handle the situation immediately, but with a sensitive and tactful approach.

Option C: In view of this Option C is not appropriate. If he is hungover his judgement is likely to be impaired and patient safety may be at risk. Thus to do nothing is not an option.

Options A and G: These options are a little over the top. This is not showing any sensitivity at all for our colleague and is unnecessary if we can deal with the situation ourselves. Our colleague had too much to drink at the mess party which occurred when he was off duty. Although he should have exercised constraint when he had work the next day it seems extreme to contact the GMC or our Consultant over this. As there are other more appropriate actions that can be taken, which involve dealing with the situation tactfully, without the need to involve the Consultant or any external agencies. These options are therefore inappropriate.

Option B: This seems to be a sensitive and tactful option. By taking our colleague aside and gently telling them that perhaps it is not best for them to be on the wards and why, we are avoiding any patient safety issue and are likely to protect our colleague from getting into serious trouble. Obviously, someone will need to cover, and thus by suggesting they inform medical staffing that they are not able to cover their shift you are protecting patients, by ensuring there is adequate cover for the day if needed.

Option E: This is certainly over the top and assumes the worst of your colleague. There is no evidence from the information provided that your colleague has a drinking problem, and the fact that he got drunk at the mess party should not be extrapolated to mean he is an alcoholic. Thus Option E is not appropriate.

Option F: As we have decided that your colleague should not continue their shift, asking them to hand over any immediate jobs is appropriate. You may not get someone else to cover for a while and thus you should take steps to ensure that any immediate patient issues are dealt with. Thus Option F is an appropriate action to take.

Option D: Obviously having a mess party during the working week was not a good idea. However, your colleague should have been more responsible and ensured that they were fit to work their shift the following day. Although, you do not want to reprimand your colleague, it may be sensible to just delicately inform them that perhaps next time they should stop drinking a little earlier. It does not deal with the situation immediately at hand (unlike Options B and F) but is a lot better than accusing them of being an alcoholic or involving your seniors. Thus Option D seems reasonable, especially as the other options are less appropriate.

This means Options B, D and F are the most appropriate actions.

Question 32
Answer: D E and G
This is a sensitive issue where a colleague has come to you on a personal level to confide some very sensitive information. She is probably very vulnerable and may be looking for advice from you. However, you do have a duty to

protect patients should there be an issue. In this scenario, a medical ward nurse is very unlikely to be involved in any exposure prone procedures, however if she ignores the issue and refuses to get tested this may be seen as breaching her duty of care to her patients. However, this really is not the issue at hand.

Options A, C and F: These options involve not addressing the issue at all and doing nothing. As a medical professional this is not ethical. You should at least try and discuss the test with her, as her health will be at risk if she ignores the situation. She is at high risk of HIV and the sooner she gains her diagnosis and starts treatment the better for her. Thus regardless as to whether she may put the patients at risk or not you should at least give her sound health advice for her own benefit. Although you may feel out of your depth in this situation, to do absolutely nothing is not appropriate in view of the other options. Option F where you tell her that she is unlikely to test positive is not only wrong in view of the fact that you are not dealing with the issue but is also factually incorrect. You cannot say for certain that she would test negative.

Option D: This is a more suitable option. Here you are recognising the impact an HIV-positive diagnosis would have on her health and are advising her as a healthcare professional to get tested. Thus Option D is appropriate.

Option G: This is similar to Option D, in that you realise the severity of the situation on her health should she be HIV-positive. However, as you may feel out of your depth here, advising her to see her GP where she can discuss her concerns further is a good idea. At least you are trying to help her in some way instead of ignoring the situation entirely. Thus Option G is appropriate.

Option B: Informing your Occupational Health department is not appropriate. She has not tested positive and is not involved in any exposure prone procedures currently and thus you have no reason to breach confidentiality on the grounds of patient safety. Although you may need to get further advice if she refuses to get tested and address the issue, it is not an appropriate action to take right now, especially in view of the other options.

Option E: You may feel completely overwhelmed by this situation as a junior doctor which is perfectly natural. Thus it may be best to gain advice from a senior colleague. By leaving the nurse anonymous in this matter you are recognising that there is no need to breach confidentiality at this moment in time, and are just looking for general advice. As previously stated, she has not yet tested positive and she is unlikely to be involved in any exposure prone procedures so you have little ground to break her confidentiality currently. By getting advice from someone more senior you can then determine a plan of action which may involve naming the nurse later if you feel patients are at risk. Option E is an appropriate action to take.

Thus Options D, E and G are the three most appropriate actions to take.

Question 33
Answer: 1.B 2.E 3.A 4.D 5.C

This question is yet another scenario that tests our relationships with colleagues and addresses conduct issues with colleagues. Using our usual approach to the question we can identify that there is an issue at hand and that it is both a legal issue and potentially a patient safety issue (as our colleague may be working with children). We also have quite conclusive evidence as we have witnessed it first hand, although there may be an alternative explanation.

Option C: To make a joke about it and forget about this issue is not an option. This is potentially a serious matter and as it involves both a legal and potential safety issue it must be addressed. Thus Option C is the least appropriate action.

We have established that we need to address the issue. As reiterated numerous times it is best practice to deal with the matter locally starting with a suitable person lower down the hierarchy before dealing with a very senior authority or outside agency.

Option D: In view of this, even though child pornography is illegal, going to the police has to be the 2nd least appropriate action. This is not because it is unsuitable to get the police involved but at this stage is probably not the most appropriate thing to do. You will probably be out of your depth in calling the police as a junior, and it makes more logical sense to involve a senior who could then call the police if necessary, once more information had been gathered.

Options B and E: These can be ranked in order quite simply by using the person lower down the hierarchy as the most appropriate person to approach first. Your Consultant should therefore be contacted before involving the Clinical Director. Not only is this approach suggested by the GMC but makes more logical sense as your Consultant is likely to be more readily approachable and available. Thus Option B is the most appropriate action to take first and then Option E.

Option A: The confusing issue now is to think about where to rank Option A. We stated in Chapter 2 that when we are answering questions involving the conduct of colleagues we should try to avoid any actions that involve criticising or confronting the colleague. In this situation, to confront your colleague on the ward in front of others is likely to cause more harm than good. If you are wrong you would have made a huge mistake and even if you are correct it is likely to cause a huge uproar on the ward and upset a lot of staff and patients. Therefore it makes more sense to discuss this matter locally with those working in the hospital who can deal with the situation professionally (Options B and E) than to confront your colleague on the ward. In view of the severity of the outcome from calling the police, especially if you are wrong, it is slightly better to confront the colleague rather than to call the police. It is also preferable to doing nothing. Hence Option A is the third most appropriate action and Option E is the 2nd most appropriate action.

Partial mark answer

The only confusion when answering this question which may lead to a different ranking should be regarding where to rank Option A. This is because there is clear guidance on how we should deal with this situation as discussed previously and the other options are fairly straightforward. However, the ranking of Option A can be open to some interpretation. It should however, be ranked above doing nothing, and thus it is not appropriate to have it as your least appropriate answer, and you will score no marks for this.

However, had you ranked it after contacting the police (i.e. BEDAC), feeling it was worse to bring this matter to the attention of the whole ward; you would have scored some marks. However, as stated before contacting the police is likely to lead to a serious outcome and should be reserved until you have a little more information. Thus, although it is not appropriate to confront your colleague on the ward, and this may potentially cause a lot of trouble especially if you had got things wrong, it is better than calling the police as the outcome from this is likely to be even worse.

Similarly had you chosen to confront your colleague before informing your Consultant or Clinical Director (ABEDC/BAEDC), you would have also been given some marks for ranking the other options correctly. However, as we stated in Chapter 2 you should avoid any answers that involve confronting your colleagues directly if there are more appropriate options available. As confronting your colleague is unlikely to deal with the matter which is extremely serious, it is better to inform someone senior within the hospital that can do something about it. In addition, as there are only two options (D and C) that could be potentially worse than confronting your colleague, as they could lead to an even more adverse outcome, you should understand why Option A should be the 3rd most appropriate option in the model answer.

Question 34
Answer: C, E and G

This question assesses your ability to problem solve and also your communication skills. It is a difficult scenario and one could have a long debate on whether Page 3 of *The Sun* constitutes adult pornography or not. Thankfully the answer to this is not needed to choose the most appropriate actions. Once again we need to ask ourselves two questions: is there an issue that needs dealing with and is there a patient safety issue. We also need to ask ourselves whether we have conclusive evidence that an offence has been committed.

Obviously there is an issue as we have an upset patient and we should try to address that. There is not however a patient safety issue or a legal issue and therefore it may be acceptable to do nothing if there are no other suitable options. Although our colleague may have indeed been looking at the photos on Page 3 he may also have been reading an article on the page, and thus we need to act appropriately in view of this and not overreact.

Option F: This is entirely inappropriate as this is not a criminal offence and seems very extreme in view of the alleged offence.

Option D: This is also entirely inappropriate for two reasons. One, because we cannot truly say our colleague has committed a serious offence worthy of involving the GMC, but also because we should try and deal with any such issues locally in the first instance. Thus Option D is inappropriate.

Option A: As stated previously one could debate endlessly on whether reading Page 3 of *The Sun* can be seen as adult pornography. However, regardless of whether we feel it is or not to tell the patient off is completely unacceptable. Although, reading Page 3 it is not an offence, one can understand how it may be deemed offensive and it is not appropriate to criticise the patient and call them 'ridiculous'. Thus Option A is not appropriate.

Option E: This seems like a sensible approach to take. There is no harm in apologising to the patient on behalf of your colleague. An apology is not an admission of guilt and is likely to calm the patient down and is the decent thing to do. By telling the patient you will discuss the matter with your colleague you are at least shown to be taking her concerns seriously and may diffuse the situation from getting out of hand. Thus Option E is appropriate.

Option G: On a similar note Option G also seems sensible. Although, you acknowledge that this incident may have been completely innocent, a patient is upset and may make a complaint. It is common courtesy both to the patient and to your colleague, to inform them of what has happened. By suggesting to your colleague he apologise, it does not mean that you are accusing him of anything or feel he is guilty. However, it may prevent the matter from escalating and indeed it shows professional courtesy to apologise to an upset patient even if the complaint is unwarranted.

Options B and C: You are now left with two remaining options. One involves doing nothing and the other involves going immediately to a senior. As stated when first discussing this question; although a patient is upset there is no legal or patient safety issue here. Therefore we need to weigh up the pros and cons of each action in view of the offence. Although, the patient has obviously been offended by what she has seen, we have no conclusive evidence our colleague did anything wrong. Thus although, we may feel that we should address the issue in view of a patient making a complaint, it is more appropriate to do nothing in this situation that to go to a senior immediately and make a formal complaint. Thus Option C is more appropriate than Option B and therefore Option C is the third appropriate action to take.

This leaves Options C, E and G as the three most appropriate actions to take.

Partial Marks
As stated in the introduction the closer your answer to the model answer the more marks you will score. Hopefully it is obvious to you all why Options E and G are appropriate. Some of you may have selected Option B (going to a senior) as appropriate instead of doing nothing. You will obviously gain marks for selecting the other options correctly but this approach will not gain you full marks. Although the patient is upset you have very little evidence, if at all, that your colleague has done anything wrong to involve a senior member.

Question 35
Answer: A and C
This question assesses your ability to problem solve in a pressured situation. You have a patient who looks unwell and who speaks absolutely no English at

all. Obviously chest pain could represent a variety of things including completely benign pathology but without a detailed history you are unable to tell what you are likely to be dealing with. You have two real choices here: either assume the worst and refer or attempt to take a history at some point to see if you can narrow the diagnosis down.

Although it may not be best practice to refer with little information, there is a potential patient safety issue here. Thus personal pride must be set aside and you must treat this seriously, especially as the patient also looks unwell. You must ensure that the patient's safety comes first and that the matter is dealt with swiftly.

Option D: In view of this telling the patient to rebook with an interpreter is completely inappropriate. This patient may be having a cardiac event and to ask them to rebook at a later date would be negligible. This is not an option.

Option A: Conducting an ECG may give you some information as to what is wrong with the patient (e.g. are they experiencing an ST elevation MI) and therefore seems like a reasonable place to start. It is likely to give you more information than any attempts to obtain a history from a patient who speaks no English, and at least if you have to refer without a history you should have at least conducted an ECG that may reveal some important information. Thus Option A is an appropriate action to take.

Option B: Obtaining a history by trying to communicate to the patient with pictures and diagrams may be beneficial in a situation where there is no possible immediate medical emergency. To waste time trying to do this when it may prove futile is not appropriate in this case. In the time that you will spend trying to achieve this, the patient could seriously deteriorate and if you obtain no information at the end of this attempt you are right back where you started. Thus Option B is not appropriate, especially in view of other more appropriate actions.

Option C: Although credible, calling an ambulance may seem slightly drastic when you are not left with many options. The patient does look unwell and even if the ECG is normal it does not exclude a cardiac event. Thus unless you are able to obtain an adequate history from this patient that would indicate an emergency is unlikely you need to be cautious. We have already stated that wasting time trying to communicate with pictures is unlikely to be successful and we may be putting the patient at risk by doing so. Thus you will have to call an ambulance based on what you have before you: an unwell patient with chest pain which really is enough reason in itself. Thus Option C is appropriate.

Option E: Telling the patient to go to A&E is similar to Option C in that you acknowledge the patient needs to be referred even with the limited information you have. However, as you need to pick the two most appropriate actions it is more appropriate to call an ambulance, in case the patient deteriorates on their way to the hospital. Indeed if you suspected a coronary event and you allowed the patient to make their own way to hospital and something happened you could be held liable. Also as the patient does not understand English you cannot be sure that they would understand your instructions. Thus Option E is not appropriate in view of the fact that there are more appropriate options.

This leaves us with Options A and C being the two most appropriate actions.

Question 36
Answer: 1.B 2.D 3.A 4.C 5.E
This scenario represents a difficult situation where you need to balance your duty of care to your patient against your duty to refer appropriately and to be fair to your colleagues. This patient may be quite demanding and as you can identify little wrong with them you may get quite easily frustrated. However, you should try not to let your own personal feelings cloud your duty of care. The GMC publication Good Medical Practice states that in providing good clinical care you must respect patients' right to seek a second opinion and also refer a patient when you feel it is in their best interest. This patient is obviously very anxious and it may be in their best interest to be reassured by another practitioner even a cardiologist. However, you do need to refer appropriately and must be honest in doing so and simply not 'palm the patient off' to make your life easier.

Option A: Although you would be well within your right to inform the patient that their GP can refer them to a cardiologist, to do so in the first instance is not dealing with the situation immediately and is also showing poor teamwork. The patient wishes to be seen immediately so you are not alleviating their concerns currently and are simply deferring the matter. Also as you are the person who has conducted all of the investigations you are in a better position to reassure them than their GP. Thus Option A is sensible but should not be your first option.

Option B: This shows good communication and empathy and may also alleviate the patient's need for a referral to cardiology. As the patient has had numerous tests a referral to cardiology is unlikely to be necessary. Thus you should at least attempt to alleviate the patient's concerns before simply referring them on. Although they are entitled to seek a second opinion, by simply taking the time to explain what the tests have found you may alleviate the need to involve another colleague. Thus Option B is the most appropriate action and seems a sensible place to start.

Option D: This seems like a sensible action to take if Option B does not work. The patient is entitled to a second opinion and being reassured by a more senior colleague may help to put their mind at rest. However, to request the on call doctor to see the patient when they are unlikely to find anything wrong with the patient, does not show good teamwork. Neither does referring the patient back to their GP and passing the responsibility onto them. However, it may be your only option should other measures fail. Thus it seems sensible before referring the patient onto anyone to let them gain a second opinion from someone more senior within your department. Thus Option D is the 2nd most appropriate action.

You are now left with three options all of which involve referring the patient onto another doctor; their GP, a psychiatrist and the on call doctor.

Option E: This option however involves lying to the on call doctor in order to get them to see the patient. This approach is obviously dishonest and shows poor teamwork. Although the patient may be satisfied by being seen today, to lie to your colleague is not acceptable. As this option involves dishonesty it has to be the least appropriate action of those left open to you.

Options A and C: You are now left with two actions: refer back to the GP or ask the on call psychiatrist to come and see the patient. Although, there may indeed be psychosocial issues underlying the patient's chest pain, to request a psychiatrist to see the patient when they actually want to see a cardiologist is likely to cause offence. The patient may not be aware or may be in denial about any psychosocial issues and to spring a psychiatrist on them in this manner is likely to come as a shock to the patient. The GP is likely to know the patient better and can perhaps address the possibility of psychosocial issues sensitively if they feel appropriate. They may even feel it in the patient's best interest to see a cardiologist first, if only to be reassured. Thus it is in the patient's best interest if you ask them to speak to their GP, rather than suddenly asking a psychiatrist to see them first off, which is likely to cause more offence than good at this point in time. As there is no immediate psychiatric emergency it would also be an inappropriate referral to the on call psychiatry team. Thus Option A is more appropriate than Option C. Option A is therefore the 3rd most appropriate action and Option C the 4th most appropriate action.

Partial mark answer

Some of you may have felt that as the patient has presented so many times that there was little point trying to reassure the patient yourself and may have ranked Option A as the most appropriate action (referring back to the GP) or indeed ranked Option D as the most appropriate action (getting a senior to provide a second opinion). Although this may indeed have been the case, you do need to consider the workload of your other colleagues. You have nothing to lose by trying to reassure the patient yourself, and if you are successful will alleviate the need for all the other actions so it is a sensible action to take initially. You would however scored partial marks, had you ranked Options A or D as the most appropriate action (i.e. either DBACE or ABDCE/ADBCE).

You would also have scored some marks for ranking Option C before Option A, i.e. requesting the on call psychiatrist to see the patient before referring to the GP. Some of you may have felt that this was addressing the situation immediately and would negate the need for the patient to have to see their GP. Although this may be partially true you need to think about how the patient would feel about suddenly being asked to see a psychiatrist. Also, as the patient is not acutely psychotic or suicidal, there is no need to see an on call psychiatrist immediately, and this would be an inappropriate referral. It is therefore far more appropriate for them to go back to their own GP, who could arrange outpatient psychiatry input if they really felt it necessary.

Please note that you would not have scored any marks for placing Option E as anything but the least appropriate action. This is dishonest and has to be the least appropriate action.

Question 37
Answer: B, E and F

This question assesses how you work with colleagues and again addresses the concept of whistle blowing. You have a fellow colleague who is struggling and who may pose a danger to patients. However, as his doctor you have a duty to provide him with the same care, loyalty and respect for his confidentiality as any other patient. Thus, he has a right to be offered the same support as any other patient having marital or alcohol related problems. However, the difference in this situation is that if he does pose a danger to other patients, you are allowed to break confidentiality. Again you must always inform a patient of your intention to do so.

Option A: In this situation, one cannot assume that he is a definite and immediate danger to his patients or that he has harmed a patient already. Thus going to the GMC straight away is not appropriate and you should at least make an assessment of the situation first.

Option D: Conversely, Option D is not an option at all. Ignoring the problem is not going to be safe for the patients, neither is it showing good clinical care towards the doctor concerned. He obviously needs some support and guidance and has come to you for this. To do nothing would not be fulfilling your duties as a doctor. As he is going through emotional problems and is drinking he may lack insight, thus asking him to come back if he is a danger to patients is inappropriate. He may have no concept of this due to his current mental state. Thus he may never come back, or may come back when patient safety has already been breached, leaving you responsible.

Option B: This is a much better action than Option A. Here you make an assessment of the situation and if the situation is under control offer him the same help and support you would offer any other patient. By offering him a medical certificate you are allowing him time off work to address the situation and ensuring that he does not pose a threat to patients. Thus Option B seems sensible and is an appropriate action to take.

Option F: This again is a sensible approach. Here you are offering him the same care and support as you would anyone else but appreciating his role as a doctor and clearly informing him that if he does not get help you will need to inform his employer in the interest of patient safety. You are dealing with the situation immediately, and thus it is more appropriate than Option C where you ask the doctor to come back and see someone else.

Option G: This is clearly inappropriate. Informing his wife is breaking his confidentiality and cannot be justified under the rules of the GMC. Informing his wife will not be in the interests of patient safety as you cannot guarantee that by telling his wife it will do anything to make the patients safer.

Options C and E: You are now left with two options that are very similar in that they both ask for senior help. As a foundation doctor you will probably feel way out of your depth here and asking for senior help is a very sensible option. However, the patient has come to see you and is sitting in front of you today. By asking him to come back and see someone else, you run the risk of him not coming back and the problem never being dealt with. Thus it is far more appropriate to ask his permission to discuss the matter with your senior and deal with the problem today. Thus Option E is more appropriate than Option C.

Thus the three most appropriate actions are Options B, E and F.

Question 38
Answer: C, D and F

This question looks at the aspect of consent and also assesses your empathy and communications skills. The question specifically states that the patient in question is competent, and thus you have to respect the patient's decision ultimately. However, you should attempt to try and understand the reasons behind the patient's decision and give them as much information as possible in order to make an informed decision. If they still decline an investigation or treatment, after being made aware of the risks and benefits of doing so, you must respect their decision. It is also important to remember that no one else can consent for a competent patient; the decision is ultimately theirs to make.

Option A: In view of this Option A is entirely inappropriate. You cannot override a competent patient's decision and refer them for investigations they have declined.

Option B: This would be completely unethical for two reasons. One you have no grounds to threaten to breach the patient's confidentiality by informing their next of kin. Secondly, as the patient is competent, their next of kin cannot consent for them or override their decision. Thus although you can encourage patients to perhaps discuss decisions with their family, a family member cannot override the decision of a competent patient. Thus Option B is inappropriate.

Option E: For similar reasons Option E is also unethical. You would have no right to breach the patient's confidentiality by informing her daughter behind her back. This is even worse than Option B as you do not even inform the patient that you are going to break their confidentiality. As stated before no one can consent for a competent patient or override their decisions. Thus her daughter cannot consent on her behalf and Option E is not appropriate.

Options C and D: These options represent the recommended approach in accordance with GMC guidance. The patient needs clear and complete information in order to make an informed decision and thus you should present them with the risks and benefits of undergoing any further investigations. You should also try to understand the reasons behind the patient's decision. Their decisions may be based on fear or false health beliefs that you may be able to address. This does not mean that you try to persuade them to change their mind; but you need to make sure that they make their decision based on fact. Thus Options C and D are appropriate actions to take.

Option F: Although you cannot break the patient's confidentiality by inform-ing their family and next of kin, it is a major decision that they may wish to discuss with their family. By suggesting that the patient discusses the situation with the family you are ensuring that the whole family is made aware of the situation. This patient may have a terminal illness and therefore the patient may wish to inform her family of this but also of her wishes not to have any investigations. However, you must respect that ultimately it is the patient's decision. This approach may not be appropriate in all situations however, in view of the remaining options it is the most appropriate one to take on this occasion.

Option G: This option is ageist and is completely inappropriate. Although the patient is 88 years old they may be completely fit and healthy and have an excellent quality of life. To inform them not to bother to have any investigations and that they will be denied treatment is false and unethical. Thus Option G is an inappropriate action to take.

This leaves Options C, D and F as the three most appropriate actions to take.

Question 39
Answer: 1.B 2.D 3.C 4.E 5.A
This is a complex scenario which assesses your teamworking and communica-tion skills as well as your personal and professional integrity. It also addresses issues about consent and making decisions for patients who are not allowed to consent for themselves. In this situation the patient cannot consent to being sedated and thus you need to make a decision for this patient. The GMC states that when you are making decisions about the treatment and care of patients who lack capacity you must make the care of the patient your first concern and also treat patients with respect and dignity. Thus although you may sympathise with the nursing staff's predicament you have to ask yourself whether sedating the patient is in their best interest or the interest of the nursing staff.

The question clearly states that the patient is simply wandering the ward and the other patients are sleeping quietly. The patient is therefore unlikely to pose any danger to themselves or to other patients. It would be different if the patient was aggressive and violent and could potentially harm themselves or others. Therefore if you agreed to sedate this patient it would be to the benefit of the nursing staff and would not be ethical. In addition the patients will all soon be awake for breakfast and morning medications and the night nursing staff will therefore not have long to wait before they are relieved by the day staff.

Option A: In view of this Option A has to be the least appropriate answer. You cannot sedate this patient simply because the nursing staff cannot deal with the patient wandering around the ward. It is unethical and is not in the best interest of the patient.

Option B: This seems like a sensible action to take. Sometimes a situation requires a friendly and calm voice, or the presence of someone with more authority, to calm a demented patient. You have nothing to lose through this approach as we have already decided that we are not going to sedate this patient. Although there are also other sensible actions to take, this seems like a sensible place to start as if this works we won't need to follow any of the other actions. Thus Option B is the most appropriate action.

Option D: In Option D we accept that it is not acceptable to sedate the patient but acknowledge the nursing staffs' frustration. We also acknowledge that it is not a life or death situation, as the patient is not causing any harm or at risk of any harm, but does need to be addressed. By speaking to the nursing staff and informing them that you are not happy to sedate the patient but you will discuss it with the Consultant to ensure that something is done about it for the next night, you are trying to achieve a compromise. Option D ranks behind Option B simply because if Option B works you will actually solve the problem for the night whereas with Option D you are delaying handling the matter to the following day. Thus Option D is the second most appropriate action.

Option C: In Option C we ask the nursing staff to bleep the Registrar to ask them to sedate the patient. Although, this involves letting a senior handle the situation it is not the most appropriate action. We have already stated that there is no urgency here as the patient is not causing themselves or others any harm and that the patient should not be sedated. Thus to involve a senior in the middle of the night when there is no urgency, in addition to the fact that it really is not ethical to sedate the patient, is not the most appropriate thing to do. Also it seems like passing on the responsibility as the nurses have asked you to deal with the matter and you are requesting them to ask someone else, when you know that sedating the patient is not ethical. Had the question been that you bleep your Registrar for advice on whether to sedate the patient, then the ranking of this option may have been different.

Option E: Option C however is slightly better than confronting the nursing staff on the ward. Although, they should probably be used to handling difficult patients, you should avoid any actions that involve directly confronting your colleagues. You have also not addressed the issue at all, and the next night, the situation is likely to recur. Thus although asking them to bleep the Registrar is not ideal, at least it is in some way dealing with the situation at hand. Shouting at the nurses will not benefit anyone and is likely to just affect your working relationship. Thus Option E is the 2nd least appropriate action and this means Option C should be the 3rd most appropriate action.

Partial mark answer

There are a number of partial mark answers to this question. Had you chosen to rank Option D before Option B (i.e. DBCEA) you would have scored partial marks. It is perfectly acceptable to inform the nursing staff you will discuss it with the Consultant tomorrow in the first instance as at least you are acknowledging it is not acceptable to sedate the patient. You may have felt that this is more beneficial than trying to encourage the patient back into bed as the nursing staff have probably tried this. However, obviously it makes more sense to try and calm down the patient first and get them into bed, as at least this involves doing something about the situation immediately. If it does not work you can then proceed to discussing it with the Consultant in the morning.

You would also score some marks for ranking Option C (getting the nurses to call the Registrar) as the first or second option. Some of you may have felt out of your depth in this situation and felt it appropriate to ask the nurses to bleep your Registrar immediately (i.e. CBDEA) or if you were unsuccessful in getting the patient back into bed (i.e. BCDEA). However, although you would get some credit for doing this and not sedating the patient yourself, the examiners are looking for those who can demonstrate responsibility. As previously stated this was not a critical situation where you really needed a Registrar on the ward, and you should have recognised that it is not appropriate to sedate the patient in this situation. Thus it is more appropriate to tell the nursing staff you will deal with the matter in the morning (which is only a few hours away) than to allow them to disturb your Registrar from whatever they are doing and request their presence on the ward to perform an act that is really unethical (or just to reiterate to the nursing staff that sedation is inappropriate). You should really be able to handle this situation yourself. However, as previously stated had the option stated that you bleep your Registrar for advice it may have been acceptable to rank this option differently.

Finally you would also score partial marks for ranking Option E before Option C. Here you inform the nurses that they should be able to cope before involving the Registrar (i.e. BDECA). Those of you who did this recognised that the patient should not be sedated and it was unnecessary to involve the Registrar especially to bring them to the ward to do something that was unethical and they were likely to refuse also. However, although this is an inconvenience for your Registrar it is likely to achieve more than reprimanding the nursing staff. At least then your Registrar could validate your feelings that it is not necessary to sedate the patient and the nursing staff should consider their concerns were addressed.

Question 40
Answer: C, D and G

This question assesses your organisation and planning, your teamworking skills and your professional integrity. Technically speaking, although there is five minutes to go until the end of your shift, you are still on duty. However, you do have a right to be able to leave on time, as long as you are not compromising patient safety in doing so.

Options A and F: In view of this Options A and F are obviously not appropriate. By not answering the bleep, you may be compromising patient safety and putting a patient at risk. You are still on duty and you cannot assume that the nurse would be able to get through to the on call doctor, as they might have the same attitude as yourself and not answer their bleep as it's too early. Similarly, asking a nurse to say you are not here is also putting patient safety at risk as the nurse will not be able to deal with the situation if it is a medical emergency, and you cannot guarantee they will get be able to get through to someone else. It is also putting the nurse in an awkward position by asking her to lie for you. You may also get into trouble for taking this approach as you still have not finished your shift and may be criticized for leaving the ward early. Thus we have established that the bleep needs to be answered by a doctor in case of any immediate patient emergency that needs to be addressed. You now have the options of answering it yourself and delegating if appropriate, getting another doctor to answer it, or answering it yourself and dealing with the matter regardless of how long it takes you.

Option E: Requesting one of your colleagues on the ward to respond may sound like a good option but you are being unfair to your colleague who may also want to leave on time. By making that doctor answer the bleep, it is their responsibility to respond to the call, and they may be the one who ends up staying late which is not fair. Thus there may be more appropriate actions available.

Option B: Here you answer the bleep but may end up staying late regardless. Although this ensures patient safety, it may not be necessary if there are more suitable options. Although you have a duty of care to your patients you must also have the ability to delegate where appropriate and must try to achieve a healthy work/life balance. Thus to stay late regardless of whether you may be able to delegate the work is not appropriate and there may be more appropriate alternatives.

Option G: This is a more suitable option. Here you return to the ward but hand over the duty to the on call doctor, if it is appropriate to do so. Realistically, your shift hasn't ended so you still have responsibilities to your ward. As you have literally just left the ward it is probably quicker to go back to the ward rather than trying to find a phone to call them back. If there was an emergency you would be acting in the patient's best interest by dealing with it yourself especially as you are likely to know the patient better than the on call doctor. Also, if it is something that could be handled quickly e.g. re-siting a cannula, you would be able to complete the task and still be able to leave on time. On the other hand, if it was a less urgent task that may be more time consuming, you would be delegating appropriately and at least asking the on call doctor if they would mind covering for you. Thus Option G is appropriate.

Options C and D: These options are very similar and both involve you being able to possibly get off on time depending on the nature of the call. With Option C you answer the bleep but ask the nurse to phone the on call doctor themselves if it is not urgent and with Option D you hand over to the on call doctor personally. As you are still on duty, it is preferable to hand over to the on call doctor yourself, rather than putting the responsibility back onto the nurse, who is still well within her rights to bleep you at this time. However, these approaches allow you to possibly leave on time if it is a matter that can be deferred to the on call doctor.

Thus Options C, D and G are the three most appropriate actions.

Partial Marks

Those of you who ranked Option B as one of the most appropriate options would have scored partial marks as long as the other two options were suitable. Some of you may have felt that perhaps it is better to stay back late than to ask the nurse to bleep the on call doctor if not urgent (Option C). Although you would be given some credit on your commitment to work this question is assessing whether you can achieve an adequate work/life balance. As discussed in Chapter 2, this involves delegating where appropriate. As Option C clearly states that you only ask the nurse to bleep the on call doctor if it is not urgent, it is a preferable option than to stay back late and miss your engagement. Thus Option B was not in the model answer.

Question 41
Answer: 1.D 2.C 3.B 4.E 5.A

This scenario assesses your ability to problem solve and to cope with pressure. It also tests your teamwork. It is your first day as a surgical foundation doctor; you are on call and are likely to be stressed. As several referrals have been made before midday already you will probably not want to be the cause of any additional work. However, abdominal pain may be potentially serious and thus if you refuse the referral due to inexperience, or provide the wrong advice due to inexperience it could be potentially serious for the patient and for yourself.

Option A: Based on this the most inappropriate answer has to be Option A. On your first day you may not have sufficient knowledge to advise this GP on whether the patient requires admitting or not. If you give him the wrong advice the patient may suffer and you will be responsible for refusing the referral or giving the wrong advice. Thus Option A is the most inappropriate answer.

You now have a couple of options: either accept the referral and discharge the patient later if he does not require admission, or find ways to provide the GP with the information he requires. Going to the Registrar in theatre to ask him (Option B) is likely to take time, plus the Registrar is likely to be concentrating on his operation and probably won't appreciate you disturbing him in the middle of an emergency. In addition, asking the GP to contact someone else who is not on call (Option C) is not the best action either. This is because the GP has to ring round looking for an available Registrar, wasting precious time for the GP and possibly putting the patient's safety at risk. It does not show good teamworking skills either, as it is unfair to the GP to ask him to do this and also unfair for the Registrar who is not on call. Similarly, asking the GP to call the Registrar later when you have no idea how long he will be in theatre (Option E) may inconvenience the GP and put the patient at risk.

Option D: Thus the best and most appropriate action from the four remaining options is to accept the referral. Although your Registrar may be slightly annoyed with you if the patient did not require admission, it is a much more suitable option than the other alternatives as explained previously. It is also the safest option for the patient. Thus Option D is the most appropriate action.

Option C: You are now left with ranking three options that are not entirely ideal as previously discussed. In view of the fact that the situation may be urgent, the most appropriate thing to do is to ask him to contact one of the other Registrars but call you back if he cannot get through. This is likely to be quicker than him waiting for your Registrar to come out of theatre (Option E). Asking him to call you back if he cannot contact another Registrar, is ensuring that someone deals with the matter. It is also safer than interrupting your Registrar during an emergency operation, when he may be able to gain the same advice from someone else. Thus Option C is the 2nd most appropriate action.

Options B and E: Choosing between the last two options is more difficult. Your Registrar is busy in theatre and you do not wish to bother him. However, you have no idea when your Registrar will come out of theatre and to tell the GP he must keep calling until he reaches the Registrar may be unsafe for the patient if they need to be seen quickly. Thus although going into theatre to ask your Registrar for advice when he is the middle of operating is not ideal, it is more suitable than just telling the GP to call back later. Thus Option B is more appropriate than Option E. This means that Option B is the 3rd most appropriate action to take and Option E ranks as the 4th most appropriate action.

Partial mark answer
There may be some of you who prioritised Option B, going into theatre to speak to your Registrar, as the 2nd least appropriate answer (i.e. DCEBA). As the Registrar is dealing with an emergency, you may have felt it is safer to ask the GP to call the Registrar back later rather than to go and interrupt him. Although, you would be giving credit for thinking this you may potentially have an emergency on your hands with this patient who the GP is calling you about. Neither situation is ideal, however, if you tell the GP to call back and something happens to the patient in the meantime you may be responsible. By simply asking your Registrar for advice, you are unlikely to cause any serious

harm to the patient he is operating on. However, if your Registrar was truly busy at the time you asked him, he could at least perhaps give you an alternative option such as discussing it with the Consultant or one of his colleagues.

Also some of you may have prioritised going into theatre to ask your Registrar's advice before asking the GP to call one of the other Registrars for advice (i.e. DBCEA). The rationale behind this may have been because you felt it was safer for the patient the GP was looking after to obtain some advice from your Registrar than asking the GP to bleep another Registrar which may have taken some time. Again you would not have been marked down too severely for thinking along these lines. However, although it would have been straightforward to ask your Registrar's advice if he was standing next to you, you have to go into theatre and disturb your Registrar in a potentially life-saving and complex operation. In view of the fact that this may be putting the patient on the table at risk and is no quicker or more convenient for you or the GP than asking him to contact one of the other Registrars, this did not feature in the model answer.

Question 42
Answer: 1.D 2.B 3.A 4.E 5.C
This question raises the dilemma of what to do when you are put in a position between being fair to your colleague and being fair to a patient when a complaint is made. As with most of the questions so far the management of the situation will really depend on the severity of the accusation. In this case there is no evidence in the information provided of any true negligence and you have no evidence to suggest your colleague has done anything wrong. It may be that the diagnosis is quite clear and she does not need a scan. It may also be a simple clash of personalities, a misunderstanding or perhaps there may actually be something more serious at hand. Regardless, you have a duty to listen to the patient's concerns and deal with the matter if she is truly unhappy even if you can find no evidence of any wrong doing. By ignoring the matter you can be seen as colluding with your colleague and are not instilling the patient with confidence in the profession.

Option D: The most obviously appropriate action is therefore to listen to the patient at first and sympathise. In doing so many complaints will never materialise because the patient feels that their concerns have been listened to. The patient may just be venting and simply need someone to listen to them. Through listening to the patient without interrupting you can also gauge the severity of the situation and assess whether there is any cause for concern. If this does not settle the matter, by explaining to the patient how they can go about making a complaint, you are acknowledging that they are very distressed and are empowering them to do something about the matter, which they have every right to do. Thus Option D is the most appropriate option.

Option C: The least appropriate option is to bad mouth your colleague in front of the patient. Even if you do feel she has a right to be upset this is not professional and is unlikely to achieve anything. It is also not fair to your colleague as you are criticising them without even giving them a chance to respond to the allegations. It is also likely to make the patient even more untrusting of that doctor and the profession as a whole. Thus Option C is the least appropriate action.

Option E: Similarly calling a practice meeting to discuss your colleague's behaviour is not the best option either. As previously stated you have no hard evidence that your colleague has done anything wrong, and even so, it is best practice to perhaps discuss this with your colleague on a one-to-one basis before involving the whole practice. Obviously, this may be different if a critical incident occurred but you have no evidence of this. It is slightly better however, than bad-mouthing your colleague in front of the patient as this may upset or distress the patient further. Thus Option E is the 2nd least appropriate action.

Options B and A: Choosing between the last two options is slightly more difficult. With both options you may be seen to be attempting to avoid dealing with the situation and not truly listening to the patient and acknowledging how she feels. However, it is more appropriate to advise her of the complaints procedure than to tell her to go and confront your colleague. For one, she may feel intimidated by your colleague and is actually coming to you for help and advice. To tell her to go and speak to your colleague when she is already unhappy with him is unlikely to achieve anything. Secondly, it is more professional for her to make a formal complaint if she is truly unhappy as this can be addressed civilly by your colleague and team in a professional manner. This is more likely to be beneficial than a consultation with an angry patient! Thus Option B is the 2nd most appropriate action and Option A ranks as the 3rd most appropriate action.

Partial Marks

There may be some of you who feel that to go and tell the patient to make a complaint is worse on your colleague than to ask the patient to take this matter up with them. Thus some of you may have marked Option A before Option B i.e. DABEC. However, you would only score partial marks for doing so.

Although, it may seem hard on your colleague if the patient does actually make a complaint, you do have a duty to inform the patient of her right to complain and how to do so. If the complaint was unwarranted it would be dealt with quite quickly in house without too much impact on your colleague. However, at least the patient will feel her concerns have been reviewed and that she has been taken seriously, even if the end result of the complaint is a simple apology.

Question 43
Answer: 1.D 2.C 3.A 4.B

This is a question that tests your professional integrity as well as your ability to problem solve. You are faced with a dilemma here where your duty as a doctor conflicts with your own religious and personal ethics. There has been recent guidance (March 2008) from the GMC on this matter. Essentially, the guidance states that you should make the care of the patient your first concern and not allow any personal views that you hold about patients to prejudice your assessment of their clinical needs or delay or restrict their access to care. It clearly states that:

> 'You have an overriding duty to provide care for patients who are in need of medical treatment, whatever the cause of that medical need. It is not acceptable to seek to opt out of treating a particular patient or group of patients because of your personal beliefs or views about them'.

However, it does acknowledge that doctors are entitled to their own beliefs and that if a doctor has a conscientious objection to a procedure or treatment requested by a patient they can advise them of their right to see another doctor and ensure that another doctor takes over their care without delay.

In this situation however, the patient does not have the choice of choosing another doctor to assist in the procedure, as they are now unconscious, and thus the decision is down to you. There are only two actions that seem rather sensible and would fit with the GMC guidance on the matter: Options C and D. By choosing either of these two options you would not be compromising patient care or safety due to your own beliefs.

Option D: Option D is more sensible than Option C as the GMC clearly states it is acceptable to refer on to another doctor if you have a conscientous objection to a treatment. Thus if your objection is strong and another colleague is available to take over you would be able to ensure patient care but at the same time not compromise your beliefs. However, you acknowledge that if there is not another doctor available you cannot let your beliefs interfere with patient care. Thus Option D is the most appropriate action.

Option C: This is the only other option that does not involve refusing to participate in the procedure. It is clearly against the GMC guidance to not participate if this may put the patient at risk. Thus the most appropriate action of the remaining three options is to participate in the procedure if no one else is available to cover. Thus Option C is the second most appropriate answer.

You are now left with two inappropriate actions both of which involve not participating in the procedure. Options A and B are relatively similar in that you are leaving the Consultant alone immediately in theatre which may compromise patient safety. Thus none of these are ideal.

Option B: This option however, is the least appropriate as not only are you refusing to assist in the procedure leaving the Consultant alone, you are leaving your other colleagues short of cover by resigning and are compromising the safety of the patients that you have responsibilities to. It is also very drastic: there may be ways you can arrange with the department to do your job without having to assist in pregnancy terminations. Thus Option B is the least appropriate action.

Option A: This is obviously not ideal as again you are leaving the Consultant alone in theatre possibly compromising patient safety. However, it is not as drastic as resigning from your job immediately, thereby breaching your contract and your duty of care to your patients. Thus Option A is slightly better than Option B and Option A is therefore the 3rd most appropriate action.

Partial marks
You would have scored partial marks if you ranked CDAB i.e. not letting your religious beliefs compromise the patient care and assisting in the procedure without question before asking a colleague to assist. However, it makes more logical sense not to do something against your religious beliefs if one of your colleagues could assist without too much disruption to patient care. This is the guidance provided by the GMC and in view of this Option D was the first action in the model answer.

Question 44
Answer: 1.B 2.D 3.A 4.C 5.E

As previously stated, scenarios on accepting gifts are designed to assess your professional integrity and personal values. The examiners are looking for honest, trustworthy doctors who will not abuse their position as a general practitioner and you must bare this in mind when ranking your intended actions. On the other hand, they are also looking for those with common sense who recognise that you do develop relatively close personal relationships in general practice, and therefore it may be acceptable to accept an appropriate gift. The key is, as said before, to determine what is and what is not an appropriate gift.

Although, you did refer her early, resulting in an excellent prognosis, to be named as a beneficiary in her will does seem a little extravagant. Furthermore, you must also consider how this will be viewed by others including her family. If the patient names you as a beneficiary, it could lead to potential legal complications, especially if the family complain. The GMC guidance states that you:

> 'must not ask for or accept any inducement, gift or hospitality which may affect or be seen to affect the way you prescribe for, treat or refer patients'.

Although, you may feel the gift is appropriate (hopefully you realise it is not), it may be seen by others, especially the patient's family, as taking advantage of an elderly lady. Therefore in this instance it would be inappropriate to accept the offer of being named as a beneficiary.

Options C and E: In both these options you accept the gift. However, in one of the options you accept the gift and encourage her to inform her family of her decision and in the other option you accept the gift but encourage her to hide it from them. Whilst accepting the gift is not really acceptable, to encourage her to be dishonest and lie to her family shows even less personal integrity. Also, in doing so you leave yourself more open to suspicions about your intentions regarding the acceptance of this offer. At least by telling her family, they can have the opportunity to object to the decision and discuss her reasoning. However, by asking her to lie to the family you are more likely to be seen as taking advantage of the patient and thus Option E must be the least appropriate action.

In view of the above, it would be reasonable to determine that Option C would be the 2nd least appropriate action as it also involves accepting the gift. However, it is useful to just review the other options before deciding on this.

Option B: Conversely, this seems like the most appropriate action to take. We have already stated that it would be inappropriate to accept the gift. Thus politely declining her offer giving your reasons why seems like the most sensible action. Although Options D and A also involve you declining her offer, they are not as appropriate as they still involve you encouraging her to give away money, which does not show best practice. The GMC clearly states in Good Medical Practice that:

> 'you must not put pressure on patients or their families to make donations to other people or organisations'.

Both Options D and A could be seen as going against this guidance. Thus Option B is the most appropriate action.

Option D: As mentioned before, this also involves encouraging the patient to make a donation to the practice, which is against GMC guidance. However, it does mention that it is a smaller donation than the one previously offered, and that it would be given to the practice. Thus, although it is not appropriate to suggest she makes any form of donation, suggesting a smaller donation instead is likely to be less frowned upon than suggesting she leave her life savings and estate to the surgical doctors. Also as the donation is going to the practice, it is slightly better than encouraging the patient to give you money directly and make you the beneficiary in her will. Thus Option D is the 2nd most appropriate action.

Option A: Although, you are declining the gift with Option A, suggesting that she makes the surgeons a beneficiary in her will, is nearly as bad as accepting the offer as beneficiary yourself. Although, you would not be taking the money yourself, you are encouraging her to 'make a donation to other people' which is clearly against GMC guidance. You could be seen as influencing her adversely to give her money away to another organisation, again leading to questions about your motive. It is however, slightly better than accepting the money yourself (Option C), where you would look even more suspicious. Thus Option A is more appropriate than Option C although both are inappropriate.

Thus Option C is indeed the 4th most appropriate action, with Option A ranking as the 3rd most appropriate action.

Partial marks

There is no partial mark answer to this question. This is because the most and least appropriate actions are obvious with no other alternative. However, some people may have had different rankings for Options A and D (i.e. ranked BADCE). Here you may have felt it was more appropriate to suggest she speak to the surgeons about making them the beneficiary of the will instead of suggesting she make a smaller donation to the practice. Perhaps, you felt that the surgeons would surely turn down this offer and thus it was more appropriate than suggesting a gift to the practice. Both options involve you suggesting a donation to someone else, so are very similar. However there is a significant difference in the terms of the amount of the donation. Also, you could not really guarantee she would talk to the surgeons about this matter, and it could be viewed that you are unduly influencing her to leave her money to the surgeon, as you suggested it. In view of the potential large amount of money that could be left in her will, it is obvious why suggesting a small donation is more appropriate than suggesting she make the surgeon a beneficiary.

Question 45
Answer: B, F and G

This question represents a difficult situation where you have to balance your duty of care to your patient with your duty to respect your colleagues. Again it is a question that may involve whistle blowing. It is especially difficult in this situation as the complaints are about a hospital you do not obviously work in and you have no real way to verify the truthfulness of the accusations. On the other hand, you do have a duty to protect your patients from any harm posed by another colleague's performance. Potentially, if you ignore this situation, a patient may be put at risk, if this has not happened already. However, you do need to handle the situation carefully and sensitively, especially as the nurses accused do not have the opportunity to defend themselves.

This question also addresses the issue of general practitioners being the patients' advocate. Often, as a GP you may have a patient who needs you to speak up on their behalf. This may be due to a complaint against another colleague or even to campaign on their behalf for an expensive treatment not offered by the PCT. Thus although the issue may not directly involve you, you do have a duty to protect and be the voice for your patient.

Option E: In view of this Option E is not appropriate. Although the complaint may not involve your practice, you still have a right to support the patient and help them air their views. Also as the complaint may involve a breach in patient safety, you have a duty as stated by the GMC, to protect your patient from any harm. Therefore doing nothing is not an option.

Option E was easy to eliminate. The other six options however all involve addressing the matter in various ways, so are more difficult to distinguish between. As stated in Chapter 2, when discussing whistle blowing, you should always attempt to address the matter locally and must avoid making accusations with little evidence. With this in mind the remaining options can now be looked at and the inappropriate answers eliminated.

Option A: Going straight to the Nursing and Midwifery Council is an extreme course of action. It is equivalent to going straight to the GMC about the conduct of another doctor and does not show professional courtesy. Also, as you do not have any concrete evidence, it does not seem sensible especially when there are other options that involve dealing with the matter locally and involving the hospital itself who would be in a better position to investigate. Thus Option A is not appropriate.

Option B: Conversely, option B seems a more sensible idea. By informing the patient of the PALS department you are empowering them and allowing them to voice their complaints. PALS will also be in a better position than you to investigate their complaints further. All hospitals have a complaints procedure and you are simply informing the patient of the correct procedure and letting the necessary people deal with the complaint. Thus you are addressing the matter and dealing with it locally, as recommended by the GMC. Thus Option B is appropriate.

Option D: Advising the patient to go to the media is unlikely to achieve anything at this stage. You have no concrete evidence at all, and to encourage a patient to express their views to the media in the first instance would be unfair to the nursing staff and to the hospital. It may give the hospital a bad reputation and will damage patients' confidence in the profession. It is also not dealing with the matter locally as the media are in no position to investigate the complaint at all. Thus it is not a suitable action in view of the other options available.

Option F: Discussing the complaints with the Director of Nursing may seem daunting as a foundation doctor. However, by speaking informally with them, you are addressing the complaints without going overboard. They would be able to investigate the matter further and you are speaking up for the patients on their behalf. You are also addressing the matter immediately in case there is any risk to patient safety. Thus Option F would seem like an appropriate action to take.

Option C: This may seem like a more suitable action to Option F simply because you feel more comfortable letting someone more senior handle this. Although, you would be reasonable in feeling that way, it is not appropriate to wait until the next practice meeting. This may not be for some time, and thus by delaying dealing with the issue, patient safety could potentially be breached. Thus Option F is appropriate, as it deals with the situation immediately, whereas Option C is not as it involves unnecessary delay.

Option G: Option G is similar to Option F in that you involve a senior figure at the local hospital in the matter. The Clinical Director would be able to investigate any complaints that you have. This would be addressing immediately the matter at hand but will be dealing with it locally as advised by the GMC. It is therefore more appropriate than delaying dealing with the matter to the next practice meeting or going to the Nursing and Midwifery Council. Thus Option G is an appropriate action to take.

This leaves Options B, F and G as the three most appropriate actions to take.

Partial Marks
Some of you may have selected Option A as an appropriate answer instead of Option G thinking that it would be better to involve an organisation that is involved with nursing standards than the Clinical Director of the hospital. You would have gained some marks for selecting Options B and F correctly if you had done this. However as this council is similar to what the GMC is for doctors, and would involve going to an external agency, you should understand why it was more appropriate to select Option F. Thus you would only gain partial marks for ranking Option A instead of Option G as the 3rd most appropriate action.

Question 46
Answer: 1.B 2.C 3.D 4.A
This question represents a dilemma where you have a conflict between your duty of care to a patient and your personal or religious beliefs. We have already mentioned the new GMC guidance on this in a similar question. However, to summarise again the GMC states that:

> 'If carrying out a particular procedure or giving advice about it conflicts with your religious or moral beliefs, and this conflict might affect the treatment or advice you provide, you must explain this to the patient and tell them they have the right to see another doctor. You must be satisfied that the patient has sufficient information to enable them to exercise that right. If it is not practical for a patient to arrange to see another doctor, you must ensure that

arrangements are made for another suitably qualified colleague to take over your role'.

The GMC also states that:

'You must not express to your patients your personal beliefs, including political, religious or moral beliefs, in ways that exploit their vulnerability or that are likely to cause them distress.'

This means that you have a right to object to the termination and inform the patient that a referral would conflict with your religious beliefs. However, it would not be appropriate to make the patient feel bad and give her a moral lecture on contraception when she is vulnerable and impose your own personal and moral beliefs on the patient.

Options D and A: In view of this Options D and A where you tell the patient she has no right to go for a termination as she should have been using contraception is not appropriate. Whatever your views on the situation you should not be imposing your beliefs on the patient. This is distinctly different to Options B and C where you simply say it is against your religious beliefs. Thus Options D and A are both entirely inappropriate. Option A however is the least appropriate as you are now forbidding the patient to have a termination on the NHS due to your own beliefs. This is distinctly against the GMC guidance which states that you must ensure the patient see another doctor that can help them. Thus it is more appropriate to ask them to see one of your colleagues in the practice than telling them to go privately. Thus Option A is the least appropriate action, with Option D being the 2nd least appropriate action.

Options B and C: These options are more appropriate as it involves telling the patient that termination is against your beliefs without trying to impose those beliefs onto the patient. In choosing the ranking between these two options you need to consider the patient and the option that is likely to help the patient immediately. As Option B involves referring the patient directly to your colleague they are likely to gain a referral for termination quicker and therefore is likely to be more beneficial for the patient. Being seen in a family planning clinic, on the other hand, may take slightly longer and is more inconvenient for the patient. Thus Option B is the most appropriate action as it allows the matter to be dealt with quicker. This makes Option C the 2nd most appropriate action.

Partial mark answer

In this question it should be obvious that Options B and C are far more appropriate than Options A and D, and as long as you have recognised this you will score marks. Therefore, if you had ranked Options B and C the other way round and/or Options A and D the other way round (i.e. CBAD/CBDA or BCAD/BCDA) you would still score some marks. However, you will not score many marks for doing this, as you are then prioritising the options that make a referral inconvenient and difficult for the patient such as going to a family planning clinic or having a termination conducted privately.

Question 47
Answer: A, D and G

This is a difficult situation where you need to show that you are safe and can provide good clinical care. Once again there is GMC guidance on this situation which clearly states that in providing care you must:

> 'prescribe drugs or treatment, including repeat prescriptions, only when you have adequate knowledge of the patient's health, and are satisfied that the drugs or treatment serve the patient's needs'.

In this scenario, you have no idea of whether the patient is actually on this high dose of temazepam and indeed whether it is in her best interests to be on it. As this medication is usually used for insomnia it is unlikely to present a life or death situation if she does not have it, although the patient may be very distressed over the weekend without it. On the other hand if you give such a large dose without knowing her full history or current mental state it could be dangerous and possibly fatal.

Options C and G: The most obvious solution to this scenario is to contact her GP to confirm she is actually on this dose. However, you have not seen or examined this patient and it may be perhaps she is depressed or even suicidal. Thus although you know she is on this medication, and her previous GP has felt it safe to put this on repeat, you are still responsible for this patient. Thus it would be safer once you confirm she is on temazepam to just prescribe a few tablets until you can review her, than to give her a full 28 days supply, without ever seeing the patient. Thus Option C is not the most appropriate. Option G however, is more suitable as you are giving her a few tablets, subsequent to confirming she is taking this dose, but not giving any more until she is reviewed. Thus Option G is appropriate.

Option A: Although the patient may have a restless weekend without the temazepam she is unlikely to come to any serious harm. She is less likely to come to any harm from not having the tablets than you giving her a large supply of the tablets without reviewing her. Thus Option A could be appropriate if the other options are less suitable.

Option B: Here you are acknowledging that you need to see the patient but are giving her 14 days' supply in the meantime. Although it may not seem like a large amount, if she was to take all 14 tablets at once because she was suicidal, she may come to some harm. Thus Option B is not appropriate in view of the fact that there are more appropriate options. Not giving her the tablets over the weekend until you see her (Option A) is more suitable than Option B for safety reasons.

Options E and F: Although you are not in any danger here of being responsible for any safety issues arising from these actions, you have subsequently passed this responsibility onto other services. Accident and emergency and the out of hours team are not going to be in any better position than you in knowing this patient's previous history. As it is not an emergency medication, it seems unfair and an abuse of services to refer this patient to A&E or the out of hours service. Had it been an emergency medication however, e.g. methadone, this may have been appropriate. Thus Options E and F are not appropriate.

Option D: This is similar to Option G in that you only give the patient a few tablets until she can be reviewed the following Tuesday. With Option G however, you have confirmed her medications with her GP before issuing the tablets. This is obviously preferable but you may have found her GP unobtainable or may have not been able to obtain the necessary information. In view of the other options, Option D would be a much safer option than Option B where you prescribe 14 tablets. It is also obviously safer than Option C where you give her 28 days' supply. Although Options E and F are safer in theory than prescribing a few tablets, it is not appropriate to refer to these services for simple temazepam and thus Option D is more appropriate.

This leaves us with Options A, D and G as the three most appropriate answers.

Question 48
Answer: 1.B 2.D 3.A 4.C
This question revolves around patient confidentiality and the GMC and DVLA guidance on this matter. It assesses your communication skills as well as your ability to problem solve. This is a difficult and sensitive matter that needs to be

addressed very carefully. You have a duty to safeguard the public however you also have a duty to try and maintain your patient's confidentiality and only break it if truly necessary.

All of the options involve doing something to attempt to stop the patient from driving. They just address the situation in different ways. Although, the patient is going against your advice you must try to still be sympathetic in the matter and be considerate towards your patient and their right for confidentiality.

Option C: This option seems rather extreme. You do need to stop your patient from driving, however, the guidance states that you must take reasonable steps to do so before breaking their confidentiality. As discussed in Chapter 2 this may involve having to explain why they cannot drive again, offering them a second opinion, or involving their next of kin if they agree for you to do so. By going to their employer you are not really giving them a chance to stop driving themselves without having to reveal information to a third party. Also to go behind their back and inform the bus depot is not only breaking their confidentiality, but cannot guarantee that they will stop driving in general. You would have no concrete grounds to break their confidentiality in this circumstance as it would not necessarily stop them from driving as a whole. Thus Option C is the least appropriate option.

Option A: This option again is unprofessional and shows no sensitivity at all towards your patient. As stated in Chapter 2, you should avoid any actions that involve confronting your colleagues or patients. It may be the case that the patient does not agree with his diagnosis or does not understand the implications. It would not be professional to discuss this matter whilst on the bus in front of other customers who may overhear and therefore Option A is inappropriate. It is slightly better however than going behind his back and breaking his confidentiality to his employer and asking them to fire him from his job. Also as we have already stated you could not be sure he would stop driving altogether by informing his employer and hence you could not argue that you broke his confidentiality on the grounds of the safety of the public. Thus Option C is even more inappropriate than Option A. This leaves Option A as the 2nd least appropriate action.

Options B and D: These options involve addressing the matter in a more controlled and civilised manner. The key in ordering these actions is to think of what would be the most considerate option to the patient as well as thinking about the GMC/DVLA guidance. With Option B, by asking the patient to book an appointment to discuss the matter you will be able to have a proper discussion with the patient and establish if there is any other way you can stop the patient from driving before informing the DVLA. Option D, although is correct in saying that you will have no option but to inform the DVLA if he does not stop driving, seems to be a little inflexible. This does not give you or the patient any other option in resolving the matter before having to go to the DVLA. Thus Option B is the most appropriate option and Option D is the 2nd most appropriate option.

Question 49
Answer: 1.C 2.D 3.A 4.E 5.B

This question assesses your professional integrity and your willingness to protect your patients even if it means exposing conduct issues in your colleagues. In this scenario you have already approached your Consultant in an attempt to address the situation. However no action was taken and the patients are still at risk. As discussed previously, the guidance issued by the GMC does state that if the matter is not resolved locally that you may contact more senior authorities. You do have a duty to do something about the matter even if it may involve being out of your comfort zone and approaching your Clinical Director or the GMC. You can never ignore the matter when there is a patient safety issue.

Option B: In view of this option B has to be the least appropriate action. You cannot simply do nothing. Although your Consultant may be at the top of the hierarchy within the team he is not the only person who can deal with this situation. Thus Option B is the least appropriate action.

Options C and D: As stated we have a duty to do something about this matter. As a foundation doctor you may not feel quite comfortable going straight to the Clinical Director. Therefore it may be wiser to speak to another Consultant independent of your team to ask for assistance first. Obviously if this did not resolve the situation you may need to go higher than this. As we have stated before you should try and deal with the situation locally before involving outside agencies and thus it would make sense to go to the Clinical Director of the hospital next before contacting the GMC. Thus Option C is the most appropriate action and Option D is the 2nd most appropriate action.

Options A and E: Contacting the GMC may seem drastic but if no one within the hospital is taking action against this Registrar who is putting patients at risk you must do something about it. The GMC guidance does state that you may contact external authorities if the matter is not resolved locally. Option E where you go to the media is obviously not ideal. This may cost you your job and may have severe implications. It is also not really dealing with the matter at hand as you cannot guarantee that anything will be done by this approach.

Thus Option A ranks before Option E, and is the 3rd most appropriate action. However, at least by involving the media it will bring the matter to the attention of the authorities and hopefully lead to something being done about it. Although it is not the ideal way of handling the situation it is better than doing nothing. Thus Option E is the 4th most appropriate action to take.

Partial Mark Answer

You would have scored partial marks for going to the Clinical Director before another Consultant (i.e. DCAEB). The key here is to understand that you need to deal with the issue and it is preferable to discuss it with someone within the hospital prior to taking it to an outside agency. Obviously, as a foundation doctor it may be more sensible to discuss it with another Consultant who will have more experience and authority to deal with the matter. However, you would not be overly penalised for going to the Clinical Director first.

Question 50
Answer: 1.C 2.B 3.D 4.A 5.E

This question tests your ability to organise and problem solve. You are in a situation where you are already late for your shift but have now come across an accident where medical assistance may be required. The GMC states in Good Medical Practice:

> 'In an emergency, wherever it arises, you must offer assistance, taking account of your own safety, your competence, and the availability of other options for care'.

In this situation, the police are already there and thus an ambulance is likely to be on its way if it is needed. There is no mention of the severity of the accident and it may have been a very minor incident, hence why only the police are present. To waste time attending the accident if your help is not needed, risks putting the patients in A&E at risk as they are now short of a doctor. In view of the fact that the police are already present and are well equipped to call an ambulance if needed, you do not necessarily have to attend the accident, especially as it may not necessarily be an 'emergency'.

Option C: In view of this the most appropriate action would be Option C. By simply asking if your attendance is needed you are assessing whether it is indeed an emergency, and if perhaps the ambulance is already on its way. Thus if your presence is really needed you are fulfilling your duties as a doctor but at the same time if you are not needed, you are not wasting time and putting you're A&E patients at risk.

Option E: The least appropriate action is Option E. Driving the accident victim to A&E is not safe for you or the patient. You will be in an unsafe position if the injuries are serious and the victim deteriorates during your journey. You may not be in a position to deal with the medical needs of the patient alone, putting you in a medico-legal predicament as well as compromising patient safety. If on the other hand the injuries to that person are only minor, you cannot justify being late for your shift by wasting time to transport the patients. Thus Option E is the least appropriate action.

You are now left with three options: one of them involves stopping and attending the accident and the other two involve continuing to your shift as planned. As stated previously, by stopping unnecessarily you may be putting your patients in A&E at risk and you are also being unfair to your colleagues who are expecting you.

Option A: As the police are already there, if it is an emergency, they can call an ambulance who will be better equipped to deal with any RTA victims than you would be able to alone and with no equipment. However, if it was a severe accident the ambulance would usually be present before or at the same time as the police, so it is probably a minor RTA. Thus the 2nd least appropriate action is to stop and park your car and attend the accident, delaying your attendance to A&E.

Options B and D: With regards to the other two options, it seems a bit senseless calling for an ambulance yourself when the police are there. The police are much more likely to know the status of the victims and the details of the accident and can give more information to the ambulance crew than you could as a visual passer-by. Thus, it is more appropriate to just go straight to your shift and let the police handle the situation, than to dial 999 for an ambulance. Option B is more appropriate than Option D. This means that Option B is the 2nd most appropriate action and Option D is the 3rd most appropriate action to take.

Partial marks

There are a few partial mark variants to this question. Had you ranked attending to the accident as the 2nd most appropriate action (i.e. CABDE) you would have scored some marks. Although you may be commended on stopping to attend the accident you need to remember your duty of care to the patients you are meant to be responsible for on your shift, and thus if it is not necessary for you to attend, it is more appropriate to continue straight to your shift. As asking the police if your attendance is necessary seems a more sensible option you would not gain many marks for ranking Option A as the most appropriate option, as noble as it would be.

Also had you worried enough to call an ambulance yourself before going straight to your shift, ranking Option D before Option B (i.e. CDBAE), again you would have been given some credit for your care of the safety of the RTA victim. However, as previously stated, as the police are already there, there is no need for you to personally call the ambulance as the police are better equipped to provide the ambulance with the necessary details. This would have obviously been different, if no one was present at the accident.

Question 51
Answer: 1.E 2.D 3.C 4.B 5.A

As this is a question on the performance of a colleague we can use our usual approach which starts with the question: is there an issue and is it a patient safety issue? On first glance this may seem like a very minor affair, however infection control is a very serious issue and patients may come to some harm if these procedures are not adhered to.

Option A: Thus as there is a potential patient safety issue it cannot be ignored. Thus Option A is not appropriate as something needs to be done. Therefore Option A is the least appropriate action.

Option B: This option is not ideal as although some of the patients may ask the Consultant to wash his hands you cannot guarantee this. It is not really addressing the issue and the patients may become suspicious as to why you are telling them this information. However, as it may result in at least some patients asking the Consultant to wash his hands it is more appropriate than doing nothing. Thus Option B is the 2nd least appropriate option and ranks 4th overall.

We are left with three options, all of which involve addressing the issue. They can now be ranked based on our duty to try and deal with the matter locally first.

Option E: This seems like an appropriate action to take. No patient has actually been harmed and it seems an appropriate approach to try and discuss your concerns with the Consultant first. He may simply be innocently forgetting and therefore at least, with this option, we give him a chance to try and rectify the matter. Option E is therefore the most appropriate action.

Options D and C: As previously stated, it is common courtesy to discuss the matter with someone closer to the team and lower down the hospital hierarchy. Hence it is more appropriate to discuss the matter with another Consultant than to go to the Clinical Director, and thus Option D ranks before Option C. Option D therefore is the 2nd most appropriate answer leaving Option C to rank as the 3rd most appropriate action.

Partial mark answer

Some of you may have ranked Option B as the least appropriate answer, and felt that by informing the patients of their right to ask a doctor to wash their hands it was worse than doing nothing at all. This may be because you felt that the patients would become worried if you gave them this information thinking that there may be some issue with hand washing on the ward. Although this may happen it is unlikely and would be reading too much into the question. Also as many wards have posters that encourage hand washing it is unlikely that giving them this information would raise too much suspicion. As it may result in the Consultant washing his hands for at least a few patients it is better than doing nothing at all.

Some of you may have felt uncomfortable dealing with the Consultant yourself and subsequently had ranked Option D as the most appropriate answer (i.e. discussing it with another Consultant). Although you would score partial marks as the examiners would appreciate that you feel uncomfortable, it is always common courtesy in situations like this to at least allow the individual a chance to rectify the situation before approaching anyone senior.

Question 52
Answer: 1.A 2.B 3.D 4.C

This question again is testing your professional integrity as well as your ability to problem solve. The guidelines issued by the GMC guidance states that we should not treat ourselves. This is mostly so that we can be objective and receive independent medical advice. However, if we do end up with a migraine we will be little use in our shift and may compromise patient safety if we continue our job whilst unwell. With regards to the options we are given, none of them are ideal but we need to be able to rank these options and find the most and least appropriate of a bad bunch of actions.

Option D: This is obviously the least appropriate action as it involves taking a medication that may be required for a patient, as well as being dishonest about it. As stated in Chapter 2, we must always act with honesty and integrity and thus stealing is not appropriate especially when there are more suitable options.

Option C: Calling in sick at the last minute before your shift begins is not ideal as you are now putting your colleagues in a predicament and may be compromising patient care as there may be no one to cover. Also, there are other options that may negate the need for you to call in sick, (such as self-prescribing the sumatriptan or leaving temporarily to collect a prescription), and thus Option C is the 2nd least appropriate action.

Options A and B: These options involve either self-prescribing or asking your GP to do a prescription for you that you would need to collect. Thus you are left with the issue of self-prescribing against a duty of care to your patients. Although the GMC states that you should not treat yourself this has to be interpreted in light of the situation. You already have a diagnosis of migraine and by treating yourself quickly you may be able to perform your work duties without the migraine developing. Although, ideally it would be better for your GP to do a prescription you need to think about the logistics of being able to get to the surgery to collect the script. Also you have no clue as to how long it will be before the script was ready. This means that you would have to leave work to collect the script raising the issue of cover but also running the risk of the migraine becoming worse in the meantime. Thus although you are self-prescribing, Option A is more appropriate then Option B as at least it does not involve you having to leave your shift and involves dealing with the matter immediately. Thus Option A is the most appropriate action and Option B ranks 2nd.

Partial Marks
For those of you who would have called your GP before self-prescribing you would score partial marks for marking BADC. However, hopefully in view of the previous discussion you can see why self-prescribing in this circumstance is safer for the patients and fairer to your colleagues than leaving the hospital to go and collect a prescription from your GP.

Question 53
Answer: 1.D 2.E 3.A 4.C 5.B

This is a question that encompasses two dilemmas and assesses your professional integrity. It raises issues about self-prescribing and also regarding patient safety as if you become unwell on the ward you may make errors or leave your colleagues in a difficult position with no one to cover. The GMC states that:

> 'You should be registered with a general practitioner outside your family to ensure that you have access to independent and objective medical care. You should not treat yourself'.

This is really to ensure objectiveness and must be interpreted with a degree of common sense. Thus if there really was no other way of obtaining your insulin it may be appropriate to self-prescribe. However, there are more suitable options open to us.

Option D: The obvious and most suitable option is to see if someone can collect your insulin from home and bring it in for you. This means that you do not have to self-prescribe or waste time trying to find ways to obtain the insulin which would distract you from your duties. Thus Option D is the most suitable action and ranks 1st.

Option B: All the other options involve you having to waste time and obtain your insulin elsewhere so none are ideal. However, Option B involves taking insulin from the ward, which is likely to have been sent down from pharmacy for a patient, and asking another colleague to administer it to you. Thus you are compromising patient safety by taking another patient's insulin and are also putting another colleague in an awkward position by asking them to administer the insulin to you. Hence this is the least appropriate action.

You are now left with three other options. Two of these involve obtaining a prescription that can only be used in an outside pharmacy which would result in you having to leave the hospital and one that involves booking yourself into A&E to receive your insulin dose.

Option E: Although, you may be away from the ward by going to A&E you are still in the hospital and are available to answer any calls or deal with any emergencies. Thus this is more appropriate than the other options that involve leaving the hospital grounds in the middle of your shift to go to the pharmacy to collect your insulin. Thus Option E is the 2nd most appropriate action.

Options A and C: In both these cases you need to obtain the prescription from the outside pharmacy, however the only difference is in who prescribes the insulin. In view of the GMC guidance that you should not treat yourself, obtaining a prescription from your GP is preferable to self-prescribing. Thus Option A is more appropriate than Option C. This makes Option A the 3rd most appropriate action and Option C the 4th most appropriate action.

Partial mark answer
It could be argued that you would get partial marks for booking yourself into A&E first as opposed to troubling your relatives who you may not be able to contact or who may take a while to deliver your insulin, i.e. (EDACB). However, at least if you tried to ring them first you would avoid burdening A&E, and would not have to step away from your ward duties. Thus although this approach is not the model answer it would score some marks.

Question 54
Answer: 1.C 2.E 3.A 4.D 5.B
The dilemma here is recognising your duty of care to other patients but also balancing it out with a duty to protect your own health. Only one of the options involves dealing with the needle stick immediately whereas the others all involve putting it off till later. The main thing to do in such a situation where you are torn between actions is to consider if there is an immediate patient safety issue. If there is this must always be addressed first as a general rule.

However, although you have been summoned to the ward round your Consultant and Registrar are there already and thus it is unlikely patient safety will be compromised if you do not attend immediately. However, if you do attend the ward round when you are anxious and upset about the needle stick injury you may make a mistake and are unlikely to be of use to anyone. You are more likely to compromise patient safety by attending the ward round without sorting out your own health concerns first.

Option C: Thus the most appropriate action is to discuss it with your Registrar and inform her that you need to attend the Occupational Health Department. They are likely to be sympathetic in this situation and although you have a duty of care to your patients, they should be able to manage without you for a short while. It is also very important for your own health to attend the Occupational

Health Department straight away as you may need to receive a hepatitis B booster or even take HIV prophylaxis drugs which are more effective the sooner they are started.

The other four actions test your professional integrity and the issue of consent. In these four options you attend the ward round but have varying options for bleeding the patient to check their HIV and hepatitis status. Bleeding a patient after a needle stick injury seems quite straightforward but in reality is not. You need to explain to the patient what has happened and counsel them for being tested for HIV and hepatitis B and C. This involves letting them know the risk and benefits of the test and making sure they understand all the information and are not coerced into it. Thus it needs to be done at the appropriate time, by the appropriate person and with sensitivity and care in mind. Ideally it should not be you who consents the patient, simply because you are probably not in a position to be objective, as you will be very keen for the patient to be bled.

Option E: In this option you let the senior sister explain to the patient what has happened and arrange for the patient to be bled. The nurse is likely to be a lot calmer than you and as she is not directly involved in the incident is likely to be the best person to be able to explain calmly and rationally why blood needs to be taken and ask for his consent. In fact many ward's needle stick protocols involve you informing the senior sister on the ward. Thus Option E is the 2nd most appropriate answer

Option B: Although ideally you should not be the one that has a discussion with the patient about what has happened and who obtains their consent to be bled, giving the job to a medical student is even more inappropriate. They are likely to feel out of their depth in this situation and are unlikely to be in the best position to counsel the patient due to lack of training in this matter. Thus you are putting the medical student in an awkward position and are not providing the best care to the patient, by requesting someone inappropriate to counsel him. Thus Option B is the least appropriate answer.

Options A and D: You are now left with two options that are very similar. They both involve bleeding the patient yourself which we have established is not ideal. However, in one scenario you attend the ward round and come back later to bleed the patient (Option A) and in the second scenario you bleed the patient quickly before going off to the ward round (Option D). In view of what has just been discussed you are unlikely to be able to consent the patient objectively yourself. However, you will be even less effective in gaining consent if you are hurrying to attend a ward round after the incident has just happened. Thus, if you come back later at least you will have more time to explain to the patient about what has happened and may be slightly calmer as you have had more time to distance yourself from the event. Thus Option A is more appropriate than Option D although neither options are truly appropriate. This makes Option A the 3rd most appropriate action and Option D ranks as 4th.

Partial Marks
You would score partial marks if you had ranked asking the medical student to consent the patient instead of rushing the job yourself (i.e. CEABD). For some of you, it may have seemed more appropriate to get anyone even a medical student to consent the patient rather than to do a rushed and half-hearted job yourself. Although, Option D involves rushing it is inappropriate as it means that you end up not consenting the patient properly. However, if the medical student requests consent, probably with no training in how to consent a patient, it is likely to end up the same way. He is unlikely to be in any position to answer any of the patient's questions either. In addition you are now putting the medical student in an awkward and unsafe position and making him responsible for quite a serious task. Thus although rushing the explanation to the patient yourself is not ideal it is better than putting this responsibility on someone who is not even a doctor as this potentially may have a worse outcome.

Question 55
Answer: 1.B 2.A 3.C 4.E 5.D
This is a question which assesses your organisation and planning and your ability to achieve a work/life balance. It also assesses your integrity as a person and your commitment to the team. In this circumstance you have a conflict of interest: work versus your personal life. There is not an immediate patient safety issue and thus it is feasible to put yourself and your personal commitments first, especially when asked to do something at the very last minute. Thus cancelling your dinner and letting your partner down is not an option, especially when you have been asked to do something at the last minute. Thus Option D is the least appropriate action in view of the fact that there are other alternatives. There is no reason why you should have to cancel your anniversary dinner.

From the options left: two involve not doing the presentation at all and the other two involve attempting in some way to do part of the presentation. Although, you may want to please your Consultant by agreeing to do the presentation, you need to think about whether you are in a position to do the presentation to the best of your ability. A grand round is a very big meeting in the hospital and you do not want to let your team down by being ill-prepared. You also need to think about the implications of letting your partner down on your anniversary.

Option B: This involves admitting that you will be unable to do the presentation and is the most appropriate action. In this way not only will you be able to fulfil your commitment to dinner with your partner, you are acting with integrity and allowing the Consultant to try and find someone else who is in a position to help. This is likely to be more beneficial for everyone in the long run as at least one of your colleagues may be able to help and devote the necessary time needed to the presentation. This approach is also better than agreeing to do the presentation but making a sub standard attempt at it as you did not have enough time. Thus Option B is the most appropriate action.

Option E: Although Option E is the only other option that involves not doing the presentation it involves lying and being dishonest. Thus Option E cannot be marked more appropriate than the other remaining options. Although you may feel your Consultant will not be sympathetic if you tell him about your dinner plans, it is not good practice to lie, even if you feel you are doing it for the right reasons. Although it may seem like a simple solution to get you out of the situation at the time, it does not show personal integrity and if you get caught out in this lie it may have severe consequences for you. It is slightly better though than letting your partner down and not being able to go to your anniversary dinner and risk ruining your marriage. You have already made a commitment to your partner to attend and it would not show much personal character if you broke this commitment just because you did not know how to say no to your Consultant. Therefore as it involves being dishonest, Option E is the 2nd least appropriate action, even though it would mean that you did not have to do the presentation.

Options C and A: We have already agreed that to try and do the presentation at the last minute would not be ideal. However, choosing between the remaining two options will depend on your teamwork skills. It would not be fair to agree to do the presentation but then burden a colleague at the last minute to try and help you out (and do most of the work) because you had plans and did not want to tell the Consultant that you could not do it. So, although trying to rush a presentation and complete it on the morning of the grand round is far from ideal, it is not as inappropriate as being unfair to another colleague and putting them in an awkward position. Thus Option C is less appropriate than Option A.

This makes Option A the 2nd most appropriate action and Option C the 3rd most appropriate action.

Partial marks

This question has several partial mark variants and illustrates the different ways of looking at the question. Had you felt that it was worse to make an excuse up to your Consultant than to cancel the dinner entirely (i.e. BACDE) you would have scored partial marks. This shows a high level of honesty and is completely acceptable. However, the purpose of this question is not to test your integrity (which is tested in other types of questions) but to assess whether you can achieve an adequate work/life balance. Thus although it is dishonest to lie, as the question is designed to test your ability to have an adequate work/life balance, the least appropriate action was to immediately cancel your dinner without question.

In addition, had you ranked Option D as the most appropriate answer and cancelled your dinner to do the presentation (i.e. DBACE), you would have also scored partial marks. Although you will be commended on your commitment to work, again you need to remember the purpose of the question. As the question is designed to identify the candidates that are able to achieve an adequate work/life balance this answer is not ideal. A healthy work/life balance is necessary to avoid burnout and is fundamental to being a GP. As the question clearly states that you have been asked to do the presentation at the very last minute it is perfectly acceptable to say no. It may have been different had you been asked well in advance and had time to prepare so that you could still attend your dinner, however this is not the case. Thus in the model answer Option D ranks last.

This question is an excellent example of why it is useful to get a feel for the purpose of the question and the issue at hand before answering, as mentioned in the introductory chapter. In general, most of the questions that are testing your ability to achieve an adequate work/life balance require you to do just that, and therefore not try to be a martyr and burn yourself out trying to do everything. Thus in these questions it is usually not the correct answer to drop everything in your personal life for work if it can be avoided, as admirable as this may be.

Question 56
Answer: 1.D 2.E 3.A 4.C 5.B

This question assesses your empathy and communication skills and looks at the issue of good prescribing. The patient is likely to be very frustrated about not being able to lose weight and you need to approach this matter sensitively. On the other hand you have a duty to prescribe in the best interests of the patient and to prescribe a slightly overweight patient an anti-obesity drug when it is not licensed for that patient may do more harm than good. Although you can prescribe a medication outside of its licence you must be fully aware of the risks and benefits of doing so. As a foundation doctor you will probably be out of your depth in doing so, and thus it would be safer to not prescribe the medication in this instance.

Option D: Thus the most appropriate action would be to have a sensitive discussion with the patient discussing why you feel it is not suitable to have the drug. This would show empathy and you would be offering the patient a full explanation of the reasons behind you being reluctant to prescribe it. By discussing other ways in which she may be able to lose weight you are empowering her and addressing the underlying issue. Thus Option D is the most appropriate action.

Option E: This option is similar to Option D in that you explain to the patient why you do not feel it is in her best interest to have the medication. However, you offer her a second opinion if she should require it. This shows common courtesy and at least gives the patient alternative options if she is not satisfied with your advice. It is not as appropriate as Option D as you are not really dealing with the weight issue immediately and thus it makes more sense to try and offer her other ways to lose weight in the first instance. If she seemed unhappy with your advice at that time then you could offer her a second opinion. However, by choosing Option D first you may negate the need for her to see another colleague and thus it makes sense to try that first. Thus Option E is the 2nd most appropriate action.

You are now left with three options all of which are inappropriate. We have already stated that it may not be in the patient's best interest to be put on the medication, and if you prescribe it you will be liable, especially as you will be prescribing it outside of its licence. Only one of the remaining options involves the patient not having any anti-obesity medication, and should therefore be the more appropriate of the remaining options. However, we still need to read through the remaining options to be sure that this is the case.

Option B: In this option again we do not prescribe the medication but suggest that she purchases the medication over the internet. In view of the fact that we feel the medication is not necessary and may cause more harm than good, to advise the patient to purchase it over the internet is entirely inappropriate. This is likely to come across to the patient as giving them mixed messages as if it is inappropriate for them to receive the drug, we should not be suggesting that they purchase it. Also in view of the fact that we are trying to do what is safe and best for the patient to ask them to purchase prescription medicine over the internet, where we have no control over what is being sold, is entirely unsafe. This action would be even more unsafe than giving the patient the medication, as at least then we could guarantee the composition of the medication and would be able to monitor the patient. Thus Option B is the least appropriate action.

Option A: Here we do not give the medication, but simply tell the patient that she does not weigh enough to have the medication. This shows poor communication and doesn't really offer a sufficient explanation as to why medication may not be in her best interest. It also suggests that we tell her if she puts on more weight in the future she would be eligible for the medication, which may come across as insensitive. It may also be viewed by the patient that she would be better off getting to the obese stage, which would be unhealthy for the patient and counterproductive. Thus Option A is inappropriate. However, it is more appropriate than Option C as at least we are not prescribing her the medication, which we have already stated is not appropriate. Thus Option A is the 3rd most appropriate action.

Option C: We have already stated that as a foundation doctor we should not really prescribe this medication outside its license for this patient. However, as stated before, it is better than telling the patient to go and buy it over the internet. However, although telling the patient that if she puts on more weight she will be eligible for the drug, is not ideal it is safer than giving her the medication. Thus Option C is the 2nd least appropriate action.

Partial mark answer
You would have scored partial marks for ranking Option E in front of Option D (i.e. EDACB) and offering a second opinion first. Although, you may feel that this may be more productive when choosing the most appropriate action you should choose the action that may negate the need for any further actions. Thus if you discuss the matter with her sensitively and provide her with other options it may negate the need for her to have a second opinion and thus it seems reasonable to try Option D before Option E.

Some of you may have also decided to give her the medication before telling her that she is not eligible unless she puts on more weight as you felt this insensitive (i.e. DECAB). Although, technically you are within your right to prescribe a medicine outside its license, as a foundation doctor you should be very reluctant to do so. Thus in the model answer Option A ranked before Option C.

Question 57
Answer: 1.D 2.B 3.A 4.C

This is quite a difficult question and assesses your problem-solving ability and professional integrity. It is based on a real life scenario so it can and does happen. On one hand you may feel obliged to try and help the patient and not affect the doctor-patient relationship but on the other hand you have an obligation to be truthful and honest. The GMC clearly states in Good Medical Practice that:

> 'You must do your best to make sure that any documents you write or sign are not false or misleading. This means that you must take reasonable steps to verify the information in the documents and that you must not deliberately leave out relevant information.'

This situation is even more complicated by the fact that the patient was meant to attend court and had a legal requirement to do so and is asking you to verify that he was unfit to perform this duty.

In view of your obligation to be truthful and honest and in view of the fact that this patient had a legal requirement to attend court many of the responses are inappropriate. There are only two responses that stand out as the correct thing to do and that is to inform the patient that you are unable to fulfill his request as you did not see him on the day and cannot verify that he was unfit to attend court (Options D and B).

Option D: With this option you are being honest by not backdating a sick certificate and saying he was unfit to attend court, and you are also covering yourself medico-legally as there have been doctors who have been called up by judges to defend why they felt a patient was unfit to attend court. However, by at least writing a note to say that the patient is unwell today but you cannot verify he was unwell last week, you are being honest and at least trying to help the patient in some way. Such a note is unlikely to be satisfactory to a judge but the patient may be less annoyed than if you do nothing. Thus Option D is the most appropriate action.

Option B: Similarly Option B has to be the 2nd most appropriate action as it is the only remaining action that involves you being honest. It is different to Option D in that you decline to write any form of letter or document and this may come across as quite harsh to the patient. It is however, more appropriate that backdating sick certificates or certifying that a patient was unwell at a time you did not see him which is dishonest.

The remaining two options are both inappropriate; however it is now about determining which one is the worst of the two. There are two issues here, one is that you may be verifying a patient was unfit to attend to court when you never examined him at the time and the other is that you may be backdating a sick certificate which is against GMC rules.

Option C: Based on this Option C has to be the least appropriate action as you are both backdating the sick certificate and verifying he was unwell to attend court. Therefore you are being dishonest on two counts. You cannot say for sure that he was unwell last week, let alone unwell enough to attend court. However, to make matters worse you are now breaking the regulations and backdating a sick certificate. Thus Option C is the least appropriate option.

Option A: This option is slightly better in that you refuse to backdate a certificate but write a letter instead informing the court that he was unwell last week. That is still inappropriate as you have not examined the patient last week and therefore cannot confirm that. It is not however as serious as verifying he was unwell and forging a document which clearly states it must be signed within 24 hours of seeing the patient. Option A is the 2nd least appropriate action and ranks 3rd overall.

Partial marks

You would have scored partial marks for ranking Option B before Option D e.g. BDAC. Some of you may have opted to simply tell the patient you cannot sign any document or write any note as you cannot confirm he was unwell. You would be correct and well within your rights to do so. However, by at least writing a letter to state that the patient is unwell today but you cannot confirm he was unwell last week you are being honest but trying to help the patient in some way. Although this letter is unlikely to get the patient off his non-attendance it may help you to look partially sympathetic to his cause.

Question 58
Answer: 1.C 2.A 3.E. 4.D 5.B

This is a question that assesses your professional integrity and how you work with colleagues. On the one hand you have a duty to report anything that may constitute a patient being abused or at risk (whistle blow), but on the other hand you must show sensitivity when dealing with colleagues and professional courtesy. The GMC states that:

> *'you must not use your professional position to establish or pursue a sexual or improper emotional relationship with a patient or someone close to them'.*

Thus this situation may constitute a breach of that rule. If you are wrong however, dealing with the situation incorrectly may affect the career of another individual. Therefore it may be a situation where you feel out of your depth. As mentioned in Chapter 2, this is a situation where you have a responsibility to not ignore what you have heard, but you are not obliged to deal with such a large problem alone.

Option C: Thus the most appropriate actions out of all of the options is Option C. This is because you are acknowledging what you have heard but are trying to deal with the matter locally first, before involving external authorities. This approach is suggested by the GMC, and they will want to know that the matter has been addressed locally before they are involved. By discussing it with a senior colleague, you are sharing the situation with someone much better equipped to deal with the situation than yourself and are recognising when you are out of your depth. It is a more suitable option than confronting the Registrar or the patient which is unlikely to be beneficial.

Option B: Conversely, this is the least appropriate action. Going straight to the GMC when you have only overheard a conversation and have no idea if what you heard was correct or if the nature of the relationship is not appropriate at all. To go to the GMC before establishing the facts, or dealing with the matter locally, is not ideal, and as mentioned before should really always be the last resort. If you are wrong about what you have heard such an approach may have serious consequences. As this option is likely to have the most adverse outcome this is the least appropriate option.

You are now left with three options: one of which involves confronting the Registrar on the ward where potentially others may hear, another involves asking others on the ward whether they know anything about the relationship and the final option is confronting the patient and telling her she is in the wrong for having a sexual relationship. None of these are obviously ideal. Confronting the Registrar is likely to achieve nothing and embarrass both the Registrar and yourself. Involving others on the ward when you have no concrete evidence that there is an improper relationship may result in unnecessary rumour and gossip.

Option D: However, the worst option out of the three remaining actions has to be Option D. Here you assume the doctor is guilty immediately and confront the patient making them out to be guilty also. Even, if she and the Registrar are having an inappropriate sexual relationship, it is the doctor not the patient who has abused his position of trust. In addition, if you are incorrect about what you have heard you may have caused great offence to the patient and have now caused her to lose trust in the medical profession. This may escalate the situation resulting in a complaint. Although all the remaining three options are not ideal Option D is the least appropriate of the remaining options. Thus Option D is the 2nd least appropriate action.

Options A and E: Discussing the situation with other members on the team may give you an opportunity to gain the advice of others and establish a few more facts, but is not ideal as you are now making everyone aware of the situation, and may be contributing to gossip. It is also not fair on your colleague to start spreading something that may be untrue around the ward as you are not giving him a chance to respond to the allegations. It is also unlikely to be beneficial and is not really dealing with the situation. However, confronting the Registrar right there on the ward is also not ideal. By accusing the Registrar on an open ward where other patients and staff may hear it will be embarrassing for the Registrar and may cause distress to other patients. However, it is better than involving others on the ward as at least then you will give your colleague the chance to respond to the allegations. Also although there is a risk someone may hear if you confront him, if you go around talking about it to the whole team then everyone will definitely know. Thus Option A is the 2nd most appropriate action and is more appropriate than Option E. This leaves Option E as the 3rd most appropriate action to take.

Partial Marks

Some may have argued that they would confront the Registrar (Option A) before informing a senior colleague (Option C) i.e. ACEDB in order to gain more facts before going to their senior. However, this is not appropriate in this circumstance. This is because confronting the Registrar publicly may lead to some of the other options we have deemed inappropriate: offending the patient, having rumours started on the ward about a colleague or even someone overhearing and contacting the GMC. It would have certainly been different if the question involved discussing the situation calmly and privately with the Registrar, and indeed it is usually preferable to have your facts straight before involving others. Thus although you may score some marks for ranking the other options correctly, you would not gain the full marks of the model answer. Some of you may have also argued that confronting the patient is worse than contacting the GMC (i.e. CAEBD). Although the consequences of confronting the patient could be disastrous, especially if you are wrong, contacting the GMC is likely to have an even more adverse outcome.

Question 59
Answer: 1.D 2.C 3.B 4.A 5.E

This question is based on the guidance issued by the DVLA and the GMC discussed in Chapter 2, but there is also an element of common sense involved. You are allowed to break confidentiality in the case of anyone who may be endangering the public, as in this case, but it should always be a last resort. Thus you should at least try other options to ask him to stop driving without first resorting to informing anyone else including the DVLA. If you do need to break confidentiality, you should always inform the patient that you are doing so.

Option E: In view of this guidance Option E is the least appropriate option. This is because you are making no attempt to determine the reasons behind the patient's refusal to follow instructions and are breaking his confidentiality without even informing the patient, which is never best practice.

Option D: Conversely, the most appropriate action is Option D. Here you are enquiring into the reasons behind his determination to continue driving and may have an opportunity to resolve the matter without the need for breaking confidentiality to either his wife or the DVLA. It may be simply that he does not agree with his diagnosis or perhaps doesn't understand the effect epilepsy has on driving. By offering him a second opinion from another doctor, you are addressing any concerns he has over his diagnosis and the implications this has on his ability to continue driving. This will probably increase the chances that he will stop driving. Indeed, the guidelines suggest that you offer a second opinion if the patient does not accept his diagnosis or the effect his condition has on driving.

The remaining Options A, B and C can now be prioritised using the same approach. Options A and C both involve you making a last ditch attempt to stop him from driving before going to the DVLA, which in general is recommended. However, Options A and C represent two distinct ways in going about this. Option B however involves you telling him that you need to inform the DVLA as he is continuing to drive, without trying to get him to stop.

Option A: Although this option involves you making some attempt to stop him from driving, threatening to tell his wife is not appropriate. Although obtaining his consent to discuss the matter with his wife may be helpful, and is recommended by the DVLA, it is distinctly different from threatening to tell his wife. This is unlikely to achieve anything apart from angering the patient and will not necessarily stop the patient from driving. You do not have permission to tell his wife and thus you would be breaking confidentiality with little justification for doing so. Although you would be within your rights to break his confidentiality and inform the DVLA you would not be within your rights to break his confidentiality and tell his wife. This is because by telling his wife you could not ensure that he stopped driving and thus could not adequately argue that the breach in confidentiality was in the best interests of patient safety. Thus Option A is the 2nd least appropriate option.

Options B and C: Option C is similar to Option A, but involves obtaining his consent to tell his wife. It may be that she could have a word with him or explain things to him in a different way that may encourage him to stop driving. As stated in Chapter 2 the guidance issued states that we should attempt to pursuade the patient to stop driving before informing the DVLA, including discussing it with a next of kin if the patient consents. Thus Option C is more appropriate than Option B where we make no attempt to stop him from driving again before informing the DVLA. Therefore Option C is the 2nd most appropriate action and Option B is the 3rd most appropriate action.

Partial mark answer
Had you ranked Option C before Option D and asked for his consent to discuss it with his wife first (i.e. CDBAE) you would have scored partial marks. Here you are again trying to persuade him to stop driving, and trying to involve his wife to help you in this matter, with his consent. However, if you can deal with the matter without the need to involve others, because of confidentiality reasons, it would be preferable. Also if he disagreed to let you contact his wife you would be back to square one. Therefore in the model answer option D ranked before Option C.

Question 60
Answer: 1.B 2.A 3.D 4.E 5.C

This is a very difficult situation which tests your knowledge on confidentiality and consent as well as your professional integrity. Although the GMC clearly states that you have a duty to keep clear, accurate and legible records you also need a patient's consent in order to share their information with other health-care professionals. However, this consent is usually implied, meaning that patients normally know and understand that this needs to be done and thus you do not normally specifically need to ask for their permission to do so. However, if they tell you outright that they do not consent, this makes the situation more complicated.

The GMC has specific guidance about sharing information between healthcare professionals and states:

> 'Most people understand and accept that information must be shared within the health care team in order to provide their care. You should make sure that patients are aware that personal information about them will be shared within the health care team, unless they object, and of the reasons for this. It is particularly important to check that patients understand what will be disclosed if you need to share identifiable information with anyone employed by another organisation or agency who is contributing to their care. You must respect the wishes of any patient who objects to particular information being shared with others providing care, except where this would put others at risk of death or serious harm.'

Obviously, it is in the patient's best interest to have the diagnosis recorded and sent to his GP, as his GP cannot treat him safely and adequately unless he knows his diagnosis. At the same time you have a duty to respect the patient's right to confidentiality and are only allowed to break it under exceptional circumstances as discussed in Chapter 2. It is not acceptable, to break a patient's confidentiality simply in order to keep accurate notes. Thus you can only break his confidentiality in this situation if you feel that such a disclosure is necessary to protect the health and safety of the public. Also, as previously stated in Chapter 2, if you do feel a need to break confidentiality you should always inform the patient that you are going to do so.

Based on this guidance, the most and least appropriate answers of this very difficult scenario can be eliminated.

Option B: This is obviously the most appropriate answer. Here you are being sympathetic to how the patient feels but are explaining why it is in their best interest to have this information relayed to their GP. You are also attempting to address any potential concerns about the confidentiality of this information by telling him that it will only be shared by healthcare professionals, and he will always be asked for his consent if it needs to be shared elsewhere. If he declines despite this explanation, you accept his wishes, which indeed is the guidance set out by the GMC. It is difficult in this situation to argue a sufficient reason to go and breach his confidentiality as not informing his GP of his diagnosis poses little danger to the health and safety of the public currently.

Option C: This answer involves lying to the patient and breaking his confidentiality without even telling him that you are going to do so. In view of the GMC guidance on confidentiality and our duty to be honest and act with integrity at all times, it is obviously the least appropriate action. There are several other actions that potentially involve breaking his confidentiality, but at least with the other options you inform him that you are going to do so. Thus although breaking his confidentiality is not ideal, it is better to do so after informing him of your intentions, than to do it behind his back. Thus Option C is the least appropriate action to take.

The three remaining options can now be prioritised with the GMC guidance in mind. Only one of the remaining options involve respecting his wishes whereas the other two options involve breaking his confidentiality. There are certain situations in which one is allowed to break confidentiality which include; disclosures required by law or in connection with litigation; disclosures that are in the public interest and disclosures where failure to do so may result in risk of death to the patient or serious harm. Although, by failing to disclose the information to his GP may theoretically put him at risk sometime in the future, it would be difficult to argue that breaking his confidentiality at this point in time was really necessary to prevent him from immediate death or serious harm.

Option A: This option is not ideal as is makes no attempt to address the patient's concerns or at least try to obtain their consent to record the information which we agree would be in the patient's best interests. However, it does recognise that at this time we have little grounds to break the patient's confidentiality as not revealing the diagnosis to their GP would not really put anyone else at immediate risk of serious harm including the patient. Thus Option A is the 2nd most appropriate action, as we really have no grounds to break confidentiality in this scenario.

Option D: In this option your reason for breaking confidentiality is that you feel the patient may pose an infection risk to his GP and perhaps some of the practice staff. Although, you are allowed to break confidentiality if you feel that the patient may pose some harm to the health and safety of others, this is a difficult case to argue. The only way really this patient can pose a risk to the health and safety of his GP and staff is if they are involved in any exposure prone procedures with this patient. Although this may happen as the patient is likely to have blood tests conducted at the practice, all patients should be treated with the same caution in terms of taking measures to prevent blood exposure. Thus although theoretically you could argue that this is a reason to break confidentiality it is not really a significant enough reason to do so and could leave you liable to litigation.

Option E: This option involves telling the patient that you need to break confidentiality simply because you need to record accurate records. This is entirely false, and as the GMC states, we should respect a patient's wishes to keep their information private unless it would put others at risk or serious harm. Thus Option E is less appropriate than Option D as it is false and involves breaking confidentiality with no grounds to do so. However, it is more appropriate than Option C as at least we are informing the patient that we are going to break their confidentiality rather than doing it behind their back. Thus Option E is the 2nd least appropriate action leaving Option D as the 3rd most appropriate action.

Partial mark answer
In view of the clear guidance set out by the GMC there is not a partial mark answer to this question. Obviously, the closer your answer is to the model answer the more marks you will score, but there is really not an acceptable variant to this question.

Question 61
Answer: 1.D 2.B 3.C 4.E 5.A
This is a very difficult situation that requires some thought. The mother of the child is very emotional and naturally very worried her child will be taken away from her by her ex-husband. On the other hand we do have a duty to record accurate notes and it will be in the best interests of the child for all those who are in contact with her to be aware of the situation and the difficulties she is having. However, as she cannot consent for herself, we would have to have good reason to go against the wishes of her mother and record the consultation details in the notes. This may be for example if not doing so would place

the child at any serious risk of harm, which would not be the case in this scenario.

Option D: Regardless of the ethics of this question, we have a patient (the mother) crying in front of us. Therefore before doing anything, the humane and sensitive thing to do would be to comfort the patient. It may be that she feels guilty for her daughter's difficulties and she may need some reassurance that she is doing the right thing by getting her daughter help. Thus Option D is the most appropriate action.

Option B: We have already stated that we feel it would be in the child's best interests to have the details of the consultation recorded. Therefore we should at least try to talk to the mother to explain why we feel the details should be recorded after we have comforted her. Thus Option B is the 2nd most appropriate action.

We are now left with three options all of which are not ideal. However, it is about ranking the best of a bad bunch. One action should stand out as being the most inappropriate option, Option A.

Option A: This option involves giving the patient entirely false information. As stated in Chapter 2, we are required by law to disclose information if asked to by a court of law. Therefore to falsely reassure the mother that you are under no obligation to reveal the information is entirely false. Thus Option A is the least appropriate action.

Options C and E: We are now left with distinguishing between these two options. Option C is reasonable in that it would be acceptable to not record the information, but is not ideal as we feel that it would be in the best interests of the child for the consultation to be recorded. However, we also acknowledge that we may have no grounds to go against the mothers wishes. Option E, could however potentially be dangerous. Although, by informing the child's father about the psychology referral, the mother may avoid any potential backlash in court it could actually make things worse. You have no knowledge of the father or the legal situation at the moment and therefore it is not really appropriate to advise the mother on how to handle her ex-husband. It is however, preferential to giving the mother completely false information that the information would be safe if the courts requested it. Thus Option E is the 2nd least appropriate action and Option C is the 3rd most appropriate action.

Partial mark answer

You would have scored partial marks had you ranked BDCEA, i.e. decided to inform the mother about why you felt it necessary to record the details prior to comforting the mother. Although, there is nothing drastically wrong in this particular approach, it shows more empathy and sensitivity to comfort the mother first as you are more likely to be able to talk to her rationally once she has calmed down.

Some of you may have also had a different ranking for Option E. Those of you who did so may have been so concerned in getting the mother to allow you to record the consultation in the notes that you felt it more appropriate to try and get her to tell the father first. Thus you may have ranked Option E before Option C (i.e. BDECA). However, you need to think about the consequences of every action you take. The consequences should the father react badly to the news of the child psychology referral is more likely to be greater than the consequences of not recording the details in the notes. Thus in the model answer Option E ranked as the 2nd least appropriate option.

Question 62
Answer: 1.B 2.A 3.D 4.C 5.E

This is a potentially dangerous situation. Normally, having an independent interpreter should limit any potential problems with information being purposely twisted or omitted. However, this scenario is clearly suspicious and you cannot be sure that either the patient or yourself are being relayed the correct information. It is obviously a very awkward situation to be in and looks at your ability to problem solve. It is however a potential patient safety issue so although you may feel awkward having to deal with this interpreter you cannot ignore the situation.

Option E: In view of this Option E is inappropriate. If you do nothing and continue with the consultation you will have no clue if what you are being told is actually what the patient is trying to tell you nor can you ensure that your advice is being accurately translated to the patient. Also by playing down your suspicions and not addressing the issue, you are allowing this interpreter to continue in her work, and therefore potentially continue to put patients at risk. Thus Option E is the least appropriate action.

Option B: Conversely, as we have stated that we need to address the situation it makes sense to see if there is another interpreter available. Although this may be difficult to find last minute it is at least worth a try in case there is an immediate issue that we need to deal with. Thus Option B is the most appropriate action.

You now have two options: either end the consultation with the patient rebooking (Option A) or continue the consultation (Options C and D).

Option A: Although, it may seem safer to continue the consultation today as you have no clue if you are even being relayed the correct information it would make more sense to ask the patient to rebook the appointment as long as there was no serious medical issue. Obviously if the patient was having an asthma attack or experiencing something potentially serious it would not be appropriate to rebook. However, as the option states that we ask the patient to rebook as long as there is not a serious medical issue, Option A is the 2nd most appropriate action.

Options C and D: These options are similar in that you continue with the consultation with the current interpreter and are therefore not ideal. However, in Option C you confront the interpreter in front of the patient and in Option D you do it privately at the end of the consultation. In both scenarios, you cannot ensure that the information you were relayed in the consultation was correct. However, confronting the interpreter in front of the patient is not professional and is likely to be quite distressing for the patient, especially as they don't understand English. Thus it is slightly better to speak to the interpreter afterwards in a more civilised manner and thus Option D ranks before Option C and is the 3rd most appropriate action. Although confronting the interpreter there and then is unprofessional it is slightly better than doing nothing, as at least you will make the interpreter aware that you feel that something may be amiss. This leaves Option D as the 4th most appropriate action.

Partial mark answer

You would have scored partial marks for ranking Option C before Option D (i.e. BACDE). Some of you may have felt that if you were going to continue with the consultation anyway, it is best to confront the interpreter in case this results in her translating the information properly. This is a big assumption to take and you would have no way of proving that she had started to translate appropriately. As you doubted her professional integrity from the beginning you would be unwise to suddenly become trusting after you had reprimanded her, as this may have made the situation even worse. You would therefore still be taking a risk that you are being relayed the correct information the same way you would have been had you left addressing the interpreter to the end of the consultation. So as Option C involves confronting the interpreter in front of the patient which is unprofessional, Option D ranks 3rd in the model answer, with Option C ranking 4th.

Question 63
Answer: 1.D 2.A 3.E 4.C 5.B

This question assesses a variety of things. It assesses your ability to problem solve as well as your ability to manage others and work as a team. It also partially assesses your eagerness to keep your knowledge up to date as it involves a situation where you need to decide between staying in teaching and leaving your teaching session.

Although we do have a duty of care to our patients and a commitment to our team, we also have a right to be able to attend teaching sessions to update our knowledge and skills. The whole point of 'bleep-free' teaching is that you are allowed to have an hour of teaching undisturbed. At this time the other members of your team (e.g. your SHO) are meant to cover you, and thus you are allowed to leave your bleep with a receptionist who normally informs whoever is bleeping that you are in teaching. The problem in this scenario is that you forgot to hand in your bleep and thus you need to take responsibility for this. However, in general you should do whatever you can to remain in teaching.

In view of the previous discussion there are two options which stand out immediately as being inappropriate.

Option C: As your teaching is important and is scheduled in such a way that you should not be disturbed, to go straight to the ward, when it could even be a small query is the correct way in which to address this situation. There are other members of your team who can and are expected to cover you during this time, and you may not even be needed on the ward so to miss your teaching without even finding out why they are bleeping you is inappropriate. There are also other more appropriate options which would involve you still being able to remain in your teaching session. Thus Option C is not appropriate.

Option B: Similarly, if it is not acceptable for you to be disturbed during teaching, to ask another colleague in the teaching session to answer your bleep for you is not acceptable. It is your fault that you forgot to check your bleep in with the receptionist, and therefore your fault that there is no one to answer the bleep now it has gone off. Thus to disturb another junior colleague, who is also entitled to have uninterrupted teaching, in order to avoid having to answer the bleep yourself is inappropriate. This option is more inappropriate than going to the ward yourself, simply because it involves disturbing a colleague from their teaching, when the predicament is your fault. It is more acceptable for you to miss your teaching, as the situation is your fault, than to interrupt another colleague's teaching session because you forgot to hand in your bleep. Thus Option B is more inappropriate than Option C and is the least appropriate action. Option C is therefore the 2nd least appropriate action.

You are now left with three options: one involves ignoring the bleep and hoping that they will bleep someone else; one involves answering the bleep and asking them to bleep another team member and the last option involves answering the bleep yourself and leaving teaching if you are needed on the ward regardless of the matter, without considering any other alternative.

Option A: Ignoring the bleep would mean that you would be undisturbed in your teaching session. You could argue that the ward should know that at this time every week you are in teaching and shouldn't have bleeped you in the first place. As stated previously you are entitled to your teaching and everything should be done for you to be able to remain in your teaching. However, to simply ignore the bleep and not even answer it to say you are busy is not professional courtesy. Had you left the bleep with reception, at least they would have answered the bleep and done the polite thing to inform your ward of your whereabouts. Thus although this option does allow you to remain in your teaching session it may not be the most appropriate option in view of the other remaining options.

Option D: This seems like a more sensible action. Here you answer the bleep and inform the ward that you are in teaching and ask if they could bleep someone else in your team. Although this involves leaving the teaching session temporarily to answer the bleep, it is the professional and courteous thing to do. After all, it was your own fault that there was no other person available to answer the bleep for you. However, you also acknowledge in this option that you do have a right to your teaching sessions and that you do not need to leave your teaching session when there are others who should be covering you. Thus Option D is more appropriate than Option A and is the most appropriate action.

Option E: This option is slightly more difficult to prioritise. This option is similar to Option D in that you realise that it is courteous to answer the bleep and do so. However, unlike Option D where you ask them to bleep someone else, you leave teaching without question if the ward needs you. As stated previously, you have an entitlement to your teaching and it is important for your professional development, and you should do all you can to remain in teaching. The rest of your team are aware of this and should not expect you to leave your teaching unless it is a dire emergency. Thus, to leave teaching immediately because you are needed on the ward is not acceptable if there is an alternative option. Had the call stated that they were unable to contact any other member of your team, it may have been acceptable to leave if there was an immediate patient safety issue. However, there is no mention of this and you may be needed on the ward for any reason, including reasons that could be safely handled by other team members, or postponed.

Thus Option E is less appropriate than Option D simply because Option D involves you being able to remain in your teaching session. For the same reason, Option E is also less appropriate than Option A where you ignore the bleep. Although, it is courteous to answer the bleep, as it is your fault you forgot to leave it with reception, it is not appropriate to just leave teaching if you are wanted on the ward for a non-emergency. Although ignoring the bleep is not ideal, it at least allows you to remain in teaching, and your ward are likely to bleep someone else if you do not answer. Thus Option A is the 2nd most appropriate action which leaves Option E as the 3rd most appropriate action.

Partial Mark Answer

This question is likely to cause a lot of controversy and subsequently a lot of you may have ranked the options differently. Most of the controversy probably involves the ranking of Options E and A, and some of you may have ranked Option E before Option A (i.e. DEACB). Those of you who did so may have felt that it was not right to ignore the bleep when you were in teaching in case it was something important. As many of the questions tend to always prioritise patients first it may seem logical to leave the teaching if you are needed on the ward before ignoring the bleep. However, this question should be answered with a similar approach to answering work/life balance questions. In Chapter 2 we discussed that when we answer these questions, we must address any immediate patient safety issue, if there is one. However, if not we must acknowledge that we do have a right to have other commitments. Similarly in this question we have a right to be able to attend our teaching session and are expected to be able to achieve a balance between this and our ward duties. As the question does not state that there is an immediate patient safety issue, it is acceptable to ignore the bleep as we are in teaching rather than go to the ward just because we are 'needed'. Had it stated that a patient was in immediate danger in Option E when we answered the bleep, Option E would have been more appropriate than Option A. Thus you would score partial marks for ranking Option E before Option A, but it is not the model answer.

Other partial mark answers involve ranking Option A before Option D and choosing to ignore the bleep rather than simply answering it to explain where you are. Although, you would be given some marks for wanting to stay in your teaching session, hopefully now you understand why simply answering the bleep to explain where you are is more courteous and more appropriate than ignoring it in the first instance.

Question 64
Answer: 1.B 2.E 3.A 4.D 5.C

This is a deliberately difficult question which tests your professional integrity and honesty as well as your knowledge on confidentiality. You are in a situation where you have a 15 year old girl who is in need of medical treatment, but is worried about a breach in confidentiality. As she is Gillick competent she is entitled to the same treatment with regards to consent and confidentiality as an adult. She is also allowed to refuse treatment, if you have deemed that she is competent to make a decision. This involves her understanding the nature, purpose and possible consequences of the proposed investigation or treatment, as well as the consequences of non-treatment. As the consequences of Hyperemesis can be severe for both her and the baby, you should try to explain to her the benefits of staying and at least explain the risks of her self-discharging.

In view of this there are two options which stand out as being inappropriate. One is where you force her to stay against her wishes even though we have stated she is competent to refuse treatment (Option C). The second option is just allowing her to self-discharge without explaining the risks of doing so and the possible benefits of being treated (Option D). Without this the patient cannot make an informed decision as to what she wants to do and thus she may be putting her own safety at risk without realising it.

Option C: This option is the least appropriate out of the two as it involves going against GMC guidance leaving us open to a medico-legal complaint. The GMC clearly states that:

> 'the wishes of a child who has the capacity to decide whether to consent to or refuse a proposed treatment should normally be respected'.

Thus although she is only 15, as you deem her to be Gillick competent, you cannot ignore her wishes and treat her in her 'best interests'. If you did so and she complained, you could be at risk from a medico-legal case. Thus Option C is the least appropriate action.

Option D: As stated it would also be inappropriate to allow someone to refuse treatment without first discussing why they need treatment and the advantages and disadvantages of refusing or accepting that treatment. We have a scared teenager, who may not understand that she is entitled to confidentiality or may not understand the importance of IV hydration. Thus to simply go and obtain a self discharge form without even discussing any other options with her is not allowing her to make an informed decision. Although it is not best practice we would not be breaking the law here and as such Option C is worse. Thus Option D has to be the 2nd least appropriate option.

The remaining three options now involve trying to encourage her to stay by various methods which we have agreed would be a lot better than forcing her to stay or just allowing her to leave without any discussion

Option A: This option however involves suggesting she lie to her mother in order to stay in hospital. Although, this would mean that she gets to stay in hospital and receives the necessary treatment, it would not be professional to encourage a patient to lie. Also, should she get caught out in this lie it may make things a lot worse for her than if she had been honest about the pregnancy, and it would have been you that suggested it. However, the decision is down to her and at least you are giving her an opportunity to think about her other options without immediately forcing treatment on her (Option C) or not discussing any options at all (Option D). However, there are other options which encourage her to stay without the need to lie to her mother. Thus Option A is the 3rd most appropriate action.

Options B and E: The remaining two options are a lot easier to decide upon. On one hand you can encourage her to tell her mother about her pregnancy and on the other hand you can simply inform her that she is entitled to confidentiality and that the whole team will try their best to ensure that her pregnancy is kept confidential. Obviously her mother may still find out through no fault of our own (e.g. she may realise that she is in a bay full of pregnant women and get suspicious) but we can at least try our best as a team to keep the information confidential. If you encourage her to tell her mother however, you have no idea of the implications. She may have very good reasons behind not telling her mother other than just being worried about her reaction. By telling her that her details will remain confidential and the team will try their best to ensure it stays that way, you are being honest and letting her make her own decision. This is better than becoming too involved in the situation and suggesting she tells her mother which is not really your place to do so. Thus Option B is more appropriate than Option E. Option B is therefore the most appropriate action leaving Option E as the 2nd most appropriate action.

Partial Marks

You would have scored partial marks if you had decided to encourage her to tell her mother first before telling her that her details would be kept confidential (i.e. EBADC). Some of you could view the situation that she cannot hide the pregnancy from her mother forever and thus it would be useful for her to tell her mother so she can be supported through this time. However, although this may be the case it could be viewed as you imposing your views or beliefs on the patient, without really understanding the implications of her telling her mother. You would feel awful if for example you encouraged her to reveal the pregnancy and she was thrown out of home. Therefore ideally revealing the pregnancy to her mother should be the patient's own decision and she needs to know her other options before feeling that is her last resort. By informing her of her right to confidentiality first, she may be able to stay without feeling that she has no other option but to inform her mother, which at this point she does not feel ready to do. Thus in the model answer Option B is the most appropriate answer.

Also some of you may have ranked Option D in front of Option A (i.e. BEDAC) thinking that to suggest a person lies to their mother is worse than just letting them self-discharge without any discussion. Although lying is not to be encouraged, it is more appropriate if it causes her to stay, and is safer for her and the baby. It is preferable to just letting her self-discharge without even trying to address her concerns, especially when she may not understand the implications of refusing treatment. So although neither answer is appropriate, hopefully it is clear why Option A really is more appropriate than Option D.

Question 65
Answer: 1.E 2.D 3.C 4.B 5.A

This is a difficult scenario that assesses your ability to problem solve and your knowledge on confidentiality and child protection. Underage sex is illegal. However, in view of the fact that it is becoming more common one has to use their common sense in assessing whether to breach confidentiality. For example, if a 15 year old was having sex with a 40 year old man you may be more concerned than if it was with a 16 year old. It is also important to ensure sex is consensual and that there is no coercion. It is also important to assess whether the minor is competent to be able to consent to sexual intercourse. In this scenario however, both are minors and both are committing a crime.

However, the issue here is that the girl in hand is 12. The law states that anyone under the age of 13 is not competent to consent to any sexual activity and thus it is considered rape.

Option A: In view of this the least appropriate action is Option A. Even if you feel she was competent to enter into a sexual relationship, the law states that she is not. Thus there is no way you can ignore the situation and just give her sexual health advice. This matter must be reported even if it means breaking her confidentiality.

You are now left with four ways of handling the situation. Only two of them however, involve dealing with the situation directly yourself (Options E and D). The other two involve passing the responsibility of dealing with the matter onto the parents. In view of the seriousness of this situation, it is more appropriate to deal with the matter yourself, and thus Option B and Option C are not the most appropriate actions.

Option E: The other options involve either calling the police yourself or discussing it with the child protection lead at the hospital (Option E). As a junior doctor you may not feel comfortable taking this level of responsibility yourself and calling the police straight away without talking to anyone may be slightly drastic. Thus it would be more appropriate to discuss it with the correct person who could then inform social services and the police and follow the correct procedures. Thus Option E is the most appropriate action.

Option D: This is the second most appropriate action, as at least by calling the police you are dealing with the situation and not ignoring it. You cannot guarantee that by telling the parents of these children that they will indeed do anything about it. It is more appropriate however, to involve the correct people in this and by contacting the child protection lead you can offer more support to this young girl than by simply calling the police. Thus Option D is the 2nd most appropriate option.

Options B and C: From the remaining two options it is preferable to discuss the matter with the girl's parents rather than her alleged partner's parents. This is because you cannot be sure that this boy has definitely had sex with her as at this moment in time it is still an allegation. Thus to call his parents without knowing the facts could be harmful. You are sure however, that she has definitely had sex with someone as she has an STI. Thus, although both options are inappropriate it would be slightly better to inform her parents as opposed to her alleged partner's parents. Thus Option C is more appropriate than Option

B although both of these actions are not ideal. This makes Option C the 3rd most appropriate action and Option B the 4th most appropriate action to take.

Partial Marks

You would have scored partial marks if you decided to call the police yourself as the first option (DECBA) and felt comfortable to do so i.e. ranked Option D before Option E. However, as a junior doctor you would probably be well out of your depth and do not really have enough facts. It is therefore more appropriate to contact someone trained to deal with this situation and who can counsel the young girl and her parents. However, you would not have been marked down severely for calling the police first.

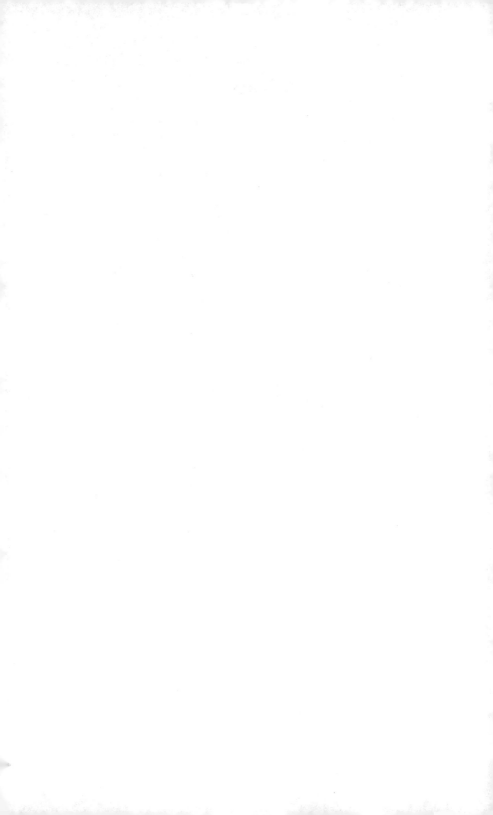

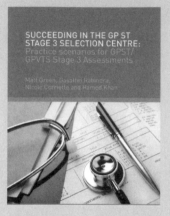
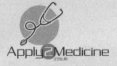